SOLACE

How Caregivers and Others Can Relate, Listen,
and Respond Effectively to a Chronically Ill Person

WALTER ST. JOHN, ED.D.

Bull Publishing Company
Boulder, Colorado

Bull Publishing Company

P.O. Box 1377
Boulder, CO 80306
(800) 676-2855
www.bullpub.com

Book cover and interior design: Shannon Bodie, Lightbourne, Inc.
Cover photograph: iStockphoto

Distributed to the Trade by

Independent Publishers Group
814 North Franklin Street
Chicago, IL 60610

Library of Congress Cataloging-in-Publication Data

St. John, Walter. Solace : how caregivers & others can relate, listen, and
respond effectively to a chronically ill person / Walter St. John.
    p. cm.

    ISBN 978-1-933503-62-2 (pbk.)
    1. Chronic diseases--Psychological aspects. 2. Chronically ill--Care.
3. Terminal care--Psychological aspects. I. Title.
RC108.S7   2011
616'.044019--dc22   2011007627

ISBN 978-1-933503-62-2

10   9   8   7   6   5   4   3   2   1

*This book is dedicated to all the
caring, compassionate caregivers of the
chronically ill people throughout the world.*

Contents

Part 2: Helping

Part 3: Listening and Observing

Part 4: Relating

Part 5: Responding

Acknowledgments

I am gratefully and deeply indebted to many people for their invaluable assistance with the writing of this book:

Wayne Melanson, director of Hospice Volunteer Services of Bangor, Maine, for his ideas and encouragement

Reverend Terry McKinley, retired minister of the Methodist church in Orono, Maine, for his assistance with the interviewing phase of the research

C. Richard Sheesley, retired director of pastoral care for the Central Maine Medical Center, for his ideas and assistance with the interviewing stage of the research

Ann Freniere, registered nurse, Yarmouth Point, Massachusetts, for reviewing the book's topics and scope

Dr. Wayne Peate, physician and faculty member at the University of Arizona Medical School, for reviewing and endorsing the manuscript

Elizabeth O'Roak, lay caregiver, for reviewing and endorsing the manuscript

Janice Gumm, a secretary at the University of Maine, for typing the manuscript

John and Rosemary Folsom, owners of the Folsom Company, for duplicating the manuscripts

Kim Morrison of the Folsom Company for logistical assistance

Robert Bull, author, for help with computer searches, manuscript review, and advice

The many health professionals and lay caregivers who agreed to be interviewed, and who completed the customized questionnaire, for the purposes of this book

—Walter St. John, Ed.D.

Introduction

This book is written for people who want to relate, listen, and respond effectively to chronically ill people. It is designed to help you understand, and be understood by, an ill person who needs your help.

This book is designed to provide specific, practical, useful, easy-to-understand guidelines for both health care professionals and lay caregivers who are interacting with chronically ill people. It offers tips about what to say and do as well as what to avoid saying and doing, and the information it shares will help you feel more confident and comfortable when you are around those who are sick.

As the world's population ages, life becomes more stressful—and as pollution increases, more and more people are becoming chronically ill and in need of proper care. Most of us have a friend or family member who is chronically ill, yet, tragically, most of us don't know how to help such people in their time of need. Because we don't know what to say or do around people who are very ill, we tend to feel ill at ease and confused around them. Fortunately, by listening and responding to a seriously ill person in an appropriate and helpful way, we can offer a lifeline to his or her emotional well-being, providing much-needed peace of mind.

There is a clear need for a comprehensive and authoritative source to which professional and lay caregivers alike can refer while helping the chronically ill. This volume is designed to meet this urgent need.

Several assumptions about the chronically ill person guide the writing of this book:

- The person's illness is serious and long-term.
- The person is place-bound, with movement limited to the house, the nursing home, or the hospital.
- The person has the ability to think, understand, and communicate clearly.
- The person needs daily help and continuous care.

All topics covered by this book were reviewed and approved by a family physician, a hospice professional, and an experienced registered nurse. However, although the contents are based on careful research, this book is not intended to be a scholarly work. Thus, an informal, easy-to-understand style of writing has been used, and a concerted effort has been made to offer practical, rather than theoretical, information.

This book's fifty-nine topics deal with most of the interactions you will have with a seriously ill person, as well as with the key factors affecting these interactions. In addition, specific "how-to" techniques are offered for each of the interactions presented.

To conserve the caregiver's valuable time, a no-nonsense, to-the-point approach is used that presents each topic concisely, yet preserves the quality and integrity of the content.

The topics are organized in a way that enables you to look up the specific information you need easily and quickly. Although each topic stands alone and is designed to be understood by itself, you can benefit greatly by reading closely related topics; you can identify these topics simply by quickly skimming the table of contents.

Many lists are provided that will help you readily identify key points, saving you time (note, too, that each topic can be read entirely in less than fifteen minutes). The conciseness of each topic allows you to gain useful information in short spurts of reading rather than compelling you to devote long, time-consuming sessions to reading.

A multitude of authoritative sources, both available online and in print, were consulted during the writing of the book to ensure that the topics were relevant and their content accurate. In addition, information has been based on interviews with, and analysis of customized comprehensive questionnaires completed by, participants who include

- Medical doctors
- Experienced nurses
- Hospice professionals and volunteers
- Hospital chaplains
- Ministers and priests

- Nursing home professional staff
- Occupational therapists
- Social workers specializing in caregiving
- Layperson long-term caregivers

Before beginning to read, you may want to consider skimming the table of contents first to get an overall feel for the scope of this book, and to see how the various topics are interrelated, valuable insights that can be gained in only a few minutes. In addition, to expose yourself to some helpful background information, you may also want to read the topics Having Realistic Expectations and Being Helpful first.

Please note that although the ideas and suggestions presented in this book have been effectively used with most people who are chronically ill, and in most situations, every person is still unique, and every situation somewhat different. Not all techniques will be effective with all people who are chronically ill or in all situations.

I wish you the best in your quest to provide high-quality care to chronically ill patients or to friends or loved ones who are ill. And I sincerely hope that the ideas offered in this book will help you comfort, and make life better for, the people who are in your care.

PART 1

COMMUNICATING

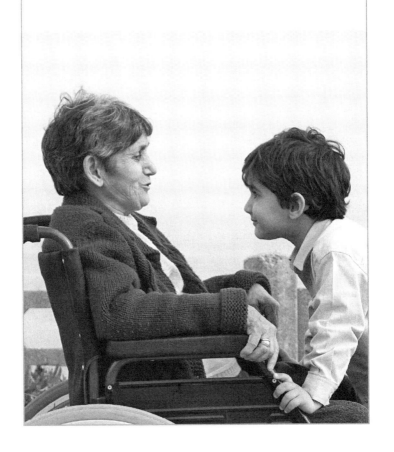

1

Answering Questions

I am not bound to please thee with my answers.
—WILLIAM SHAKESPEARE

People who are seriously ill want, and need, to know many things. Their world is filled with unmet needs, anxieties, and fears, and they will be looking to you to provide some of the answers to these questions, and to meet some of the needs represented by their questions.

You need to show an ill person that you are willing to answer his or her questions to the best of your ability. Let the person know that his or her questions are important to you, and that you will answer as many as you can.

But know when you don't know. Don't expect to have the answers for all the questions you are asked. No one could possibly answer everything he or she is asked—some questions have no answers, or only unsatisfactory answers; for example, "What exactly is heaven like?" It is also inappropriate for you to answer certain questions, perhaps because another person would be able to provide a more informed answer. Obviously, questions such as "When will

I be able to walk again?" should be answered by a doctor; and overly complicated spiritual questions should be referred to a cleric. Whenever impossible-to-answer or inappropriate questions are asked, show interest, but don't even try to answer. However, be sure to explain why you can't give an answer.

Your obligation when answering questions is to be truthful, and to do your best to tell the ill person what he or she needs to know. Refrain from saying what you think the questioner wants to hear, or what you wish you could tell him or her.

Honesty is essential. Candor, balanced with tact, is also a must. But this doesn't mean you always need to say everything you are thinking or feeling if doing so would not serve any useful purpose. When answering questions, your goal should be to get your answer both understood and accepted.

It is best not to guess or bluff when responding to questions. It is perfectly proper to say, "I don't know," when you really don't know the answer to something. It is also wise to avoid speculating. Stick to the facts—to what you actually know. The ill person is entitled to a truthful answer based on facts, so that he or she can put matters into proper perspective and make informed decisions. In most situations, no answer is better than a wrong answer.

If you don't know the answer to a question at the time but think you can find a satisfactory answer, merely say, "I can't answer that right now, but I think I can find out for you." It is a good idea, whenever you delay your answer, to give the questioner the approximate time you will get back to him or her with an answer. (It is better to give yourself a little wiggle room by giving an approximate time instead of an exact time.)

Before you try to answer a question, make sure you understand it. To ensure that you understand it, repeat the question; for example, "You want to know when your brother will be able to visit you, right?"

Pay attention not only to the wording of the question, but to why the question is being asked. Try to figure out what is behind the question. Take a minute to consider the possible consequences or reactions to your answer before giving it. Watch the person's facial expressions and body language while you are answering a question to gain clues about how the person is reacting to what you are saying.

It is important to respond to questions as honestly as you can. Always try to be truthful and factual, while also being mindful of the sick person's feelings. At times you may feel inclined to tell "little white lies," but it is generally better not to do this. Ask yourself, when tempted to temper the truth, "Am I doing this for my benefit, or for the sick person's?"

These suggestions will help you to answer an ill person's questions effectively:

- Be brief—avoid long, detailed responses.
- Speak simply, plainly, and clearly—cite examples to aid understanding.

- Choose your words carefully.
- Be both honest and tactful.
- Respond to the question asked—don't be evasive.
- Speak audibly, and with a confident air—sound credible.
- Consider the questioner's feelings at all times.
- Use *I* answers—speak only for yourself.
- When it appears wise to do so, encourage the questioner to answer his or her own questions and draw his or her own conclusions.
- Seek immediate feedback to make sure the person understands your answer.

There is an art to answering questions skillfully. And there is a right way to do so, and a wrong way—a proper way, and an improper way; an ethical way and an unethical way. The principles and techniques offered here should help you answer an ill person's questions responsibly, skillfully, and ethically.

2

Apologizing

Oh, words are action enough, if they're the right words.
—D. H. LAWRENCE

We are all wrong at times and need to apologize to someone whom we have wronged. Apologizing to someone who is chronically ill, when an apology is appropriate, is especially important, because such people tend to be especially sensitive to how they are treated.

Giving a necessary apology shows your concern for someone who is ill, and helps you maintain good relations with him or her. Fairness, common sense, and compassion dictate that you ought to readily apologize when an apology is called for.

A person who feels offended feels better when he or she receives a prompt and sincere apology; he or she experiences a feeling of relief. And people respect and admire someone who has the integrity and courage to apologize. It is important to realize that the willingness to apologize is the mark of a big person. Only a small person refuses to apologize when it is warranted.

But there is a wrong way to apologize as well as a right way. To apologize well,

- Speak confidently, without any hesitation or hint of reluctance;
- Apologize promptly—a delayed apology loses its impact;
- Get to the point—don't ramble;
- Make your sincerity clear—don't just go through the motions.

Sometimes you may sense that someone is upset with you without knowing why; in such a situation, feel free to make a limited apology. If you can't think of anything you've done wrong, don't admit to wrongdoing, but simply open the door to reconciliation. You might say, "Jane, I'm afraid you may be upset with me—I certainly don't want anything to come between us,' or "John, I feel like something I said yesterday may have offended you. If I did say something to offend you, please know it wasn't on purpose—I never want to hurt you." You can also say, "I'm sorry you're upset—what can I do to help?"

On the other hand, an ill person who is feeling irritable may say something offensive to you that he or she later regrets having said. Soon he or she may feel regretful and want to make amends by apologizing to you.

When you accept a sincere apology from someone who is ill, never make him or her feel embarrassed or uncomfortable. Minimize such feelings by smiling, acting friendly, and saying something gracious:

- "I accept your apology, and I appreciate it."
- "Thank you. I know I said some things I really didn't mean, either."

But be careful, when you accept an apology, avoid saying anything that might seem to be a rebuff of the person's apology, or anything else that might make the person feel inadequate while apologizing:

- "Oh, I don't know what in the world you're apologizing to me for!"
- "You certainly *do* owe me an apology."
- "What you said *was* really hurtful—it gave me a pretty bad afternoon."

Apologies can be a very positive thing. When made and received properly, they make everyone feel better.

3

Avoiding Harmful Questions

*A question not to be asked is a
question not to be answered.*
—Robert Southey

There are numerous harmful questions that you must avoid asking. You may not intend for them to be harmful—and they may appear quite innocent to you—but how your questions are taken by the chronically ill person is what really counts.

These questions to avoid fall into five categories:
1. Provision of help
2. Conversation inhibitors
3. Daily living
4. Health condition
5. Concerns and anxieties

1. Provision of Help:
- "Don't you realize how much I'm sacrificing for you?"
- "How can you expect me to do so much?"
- "*Now* what do you want me to do for you?"

- "You don't want to be any more of a burden than necessary, do you?"
- "Why don't you just relax, and let *me* take care of everything?"
- "How can I help you when you have such a negative attitude about everything?"
- "Why do you complain so much when I'm doing my best to help you?"
- "Why don't you try to be a little less demanding?"
- "Why can't you show some appreciation for all the things I do for you?"

2. Conversation Inhibitors:
- "Can't you ever talk about anything pleasant?"
- "Don't you know you shouldn't ask me things like that?"
- "Why do you always have so many questions?"
- "You can't really mean that, can you?"
- "Don't you realize how hard you make it for anyone to talk with you?"
- "Don't you get tired of harping about the same old things all the time?"
- "Can't you say anything without complaining?"
- "Do you have any regrets about your life?"
- "Can't you talk about anything other than your past?"

3. Daily Living:

- "What are you going to do with your personal possessions?"
- "Don't you think you could make better use of your money?"
- "Don't you think it's time for you to begin living life to the fullest each day instead of griping about everything?"
- "How can you be satisfied doing the same thing day after day?"
- "Do you prefer living the way you do, or would you rather end your suffering and go to a better place?"

4. Health Condition:

- "Don't you know you can't do that in your condition?"
- "How much time does the doctor give you?"
- "Are you sure the pain isn't all in your head?"
- "Why don't you just change doctors instead of constantly griping about how she treats you?"
- "How bad are you feeling today?"
- "Do you feel as lousy as you look?"
- "Can't you see how sorry I feel for you?"
- "Why are you always so gloomy?"
- "Can't you ever talk about anything else other than how you feel?"
- "Why do you have so much self-pity when you've lived such a full life?"

- "Can't you ever think of anyone other than yourself?"

5. Concerns and Anxieties:

- "Why do you keep talking about dying?"
- "Don't you think I get tired about hearing about all your troubles?"
- "Why do you insist on viewing everything negatively?"
- "Why in the world do you worry about things like that?"
- "Don't you think it's time to make your peace with God?"
- "Why don't you try not to talk about things that trouble you so much?"
- "How can you feel so depressed about life?"
- "Don't you know you won't get to heaven if you keep saying things like that?"
- "Why don't you try to look at the good side of things for once?"

It is imperative that you think not only about the kinds of questions you ask an ill individual, but also about his or her possible reactions to those questions. If a question won't help the situation, it is best not to ask it at all. Discretion is the name of the game.

4

Avoiding Harmful Statements

*There are those whose words frighten
more than the things they express.*
—John L. Spalding

Take the time to think before you say anything important to an ill person. In particular, you need to be careful both of what you say and of how you say it—if you say the wrong thing, or say it in the wrong way, you could create problems. Many chronically ill people are extremely sensitive, and their delicate egos can be wounded easily. It could take a long time for your relationship to recover if you hurt the feelings of someone who is sick.

It is important to know your purpose before saying anything important. Also, consider what the person's reaction will be before you say anything. After saying something, play it safe by checking to be sure that what you have said is understood the way you intended it to be.

Realize that what you say to an ill person today can affect your relationship with him or her tomorrow, and note that what, and how, you said something yesterday will affect the person's reaction to what you say today.

It is vital that you be aware that even when people are too weak to speak and appear unaware of what is going on around them, they may be able to hear what you are saying about them. Since hearing is a person's last sense to fade, be on guard against saying anything negative or critical about a person in his or her presence.

Here is a list of statements about various topics that you should try to avoid:

Your Availability to Help
- "I wish I could go to the picnic—but someone has to be here with you."
- "It looks as though I won't be able to get away for my vacation this year after all."
- "It sure is a lot of work looking after you."
- "I can't be here with you all the time—I've got my own life to lead, too."
- "I really don't need this in my life right now."
- "If you don't stop your complaining, I'm going to leave right now."
- "I have to go now—I've got no idea when I'll be able to get back here."
- "There just aren't enough hours in the day for me to get everything done I need to."
- "I have only ten minutes to visit with you today, because I've got a lot of important things to do."

- "You shouldn't keep making demands on me and the family. I'm sure you don't want to be considered a burden."

When Listening to the Person
- "Oh, stop talking like that—it's just your medicine talking. I know you couldn't possibly *mean* that."
- "I don't have time to listen to you now."
- "I'm not going to sit here and listen to you talk like that."
- "I don't know why you expect me to listen to you all the time when you never listen to me at all."
- "You told me all about that yesterday; I don't want to hear it again today."
- "I don't want to hear about your dreams—they're too ridiculous."

The Person's Statements to You
- "Don't think like that."
- "That's just not true."
- "You shouldn't feel that way."
- "You don't know what you're saying."
- "That's an awful thing to say—you can't possibly mean that!"
- "You're going to make yourself upset talking like that."
- "You're talking pure nonsense."
- "You should know better than to say that."

- "I don't know why you insist on saying crazy things like that."
- "I don't want to talk about this any more."

Giving Advice
- "Now, *this* is exactly what you should do . . ."
- "Trust me—I know what's best for you."
- "You need to rely on me to do what is best for you."
- "This is what I want you to do."
- "I don't think you should worry about things like that."
- "Don't cry—it doesn't do any good."
- "Forget it—things can't be as bad as all that."
- "You need to be brave and strong."
- "You need to have a more positive attitude."
- "Keep your spirits up—remember it's darkest just before the dawn."
- "You shouldn't expect so much from yourself."
- "I think you should . . ."
- "What you really need is . . ."
- "My best advice to you is to . . ."
- "I strongly suggest you don't do that."
- "You're only saying that because you're tired."

Criticizing the Person
- "Don't be such a baby."
- "You're acting downright stupid."
- "As I keep telling you . . ."

- "*Shame* on you for saying that!"
- "Your attitude is terrible."
- "You keep making the same mistake over and over again."
- "You're dead wrong to think that."
- "Now, you know you shouldn't say things like that."
- "I can't believe you've had *another* accident."
- "Stop being ridiculous—you know you aren't able to do that any more!"
- "You keep asking me the same thing over and over— my answer is still no, and it will always be no."

Relationship With God
- "God gives us only as much as we can handle."
- "You're going to go to hell because of the way you've lived."
- "It's God's will."
- "I don't know why you can't believe in God the way I do."
- "God will punish you if you don't . . ."
- "God has given you a long life."

Talking About Yourself
- "I've had a really rough day—let me tell you all about it."
- "I know you really don't want to talk about this, but I'd like to, so let's talk."
- "Today I want to talk to you about . . ."

- "As far as I'm concerned, the issue is closed—period."
- "Stop fidgeting—you're making me nervous."
- "You think you've had it rough? Let me tell you about . . ."
- "Don't get upset with me—*I* haven't done anything to you."
- "Please don't just lie there—I want you to talk with me."
- "The things I want out of life are . . ."
- "I've been sick, and I've been feeling rotten all day."

Talking About the Sick Person's Health
- "I know exactly how you feel."
- "Hey—things could be a lot worse."
- "You'll be a better person because of all this."
- "You look worse today."
- "I'm sure you'll recover completely."
- "You couldn't have possibly seen and talked with Aunt Molly—she's been dead for years! You must have been hallucinating."
- "I pity you."
- "I don't know why this is happening to someone like you."
- "Cheer up—things aren't as bad as they seem."
- "Things will be better tomorrow—I promise."
- "Everything will be all right—I just know it will."
- "Don't worry about it—it will all be over soon."

- "You're just going to be fine."
- "I'm afraid it's starting to look hopeless."
- "You're going to die."
- "Think positively—it may go away."
- "It will all work out, believe me."
- "You aren't as sick as you think you are."
- "You'll be able to return to work soon."
- "I heard of a person who had the same thing, and . . ."
- "The whole family is counting on you getting better, so don't let us down."
- "I feel sorry for you."

It is a good idea to stick to the facts when discussing a seriously ill person's health; talking in platitudes and offering promises of false hope can drive a gulf between you and the ill person, and can ultimately destroy your credibility.

You may intend your wistful comments to be helpful, but they may end up being extremely harmful. Remember—it is the effects of what you say that count, not your intent in saying it.

5

Avoiding Judgmental Comments

No man likes to live under the eye
of perpetual disapprobation.
—Samuel Johnson

People resent being judged by others. They don't want to be around, or to talk with, strongly judgmental people, because doing so makes them feel uncomfortable, vulnerable, and defensive. They feel they need to keep their guard up at all times.

Granted—we can't help judging what people say and do on occasion; this is part of being human. But we can strive to become more accepting and less judgmental of others. Being accepted builds up an ill person's self-confidence; being judged tears it down.

When you judge another person, you evaluate what he or she says and does as good/bad, right/wrong, correct/incorrect, and so on. A judgmental person uses the words *should* or *ought* frequently in conversation. By making judgments, you imply some sort of superiority. Most of our judgments of others tend to be negative and critical—

yet judgmental statements are counterproductive as they rarely do any good.

Judgments also involve being preachy, moralizing, making pronouncements, and acting holier-than-thou. All judgmental attitudes and statements should be avoided, because they are unwelcome, and usually create not only resentment but sometimes even hostility in the person being judged.

You can act judgmental in many ways, including through

- Your facial expressions
- Your body positions and movements
- Your tone of voice and volume of speech
- Your choice of words

You can avoid sounding judgmental by using descriptive phrases. When you use descriptive phrases, you express what you are thinking and feeling about something. Descriptive statements are your neutral observations of what you see and hear. Conversely, judgmental statements express your personal beliefs and values.

By using descriptive statements, you avoid being perceived as superior, condescending, and evaluative. By making descriptive comments, you help a sick person feel more comfortable with you, free to speak up and say exactly what is on his or her mind. He or she feels he or she can let his or her guard down without fear.

It is essential that you know the difference between judgmental (J) and descriptive (D) statements when talking with ill people. These comparative statements will help you make this differentiation:

(J) "You look good today."
(D) "I like the way you look today."
(J) "You should eat all your food."
(D) "I think it would be good if you ate all your food."
(J) "You're wrong to talk about your doctor like that."
(D) "I am concerned when you talk about your doctor like that."
(J) "You must be uncomfortable sitting like that."
(D) "You look uncomfortable when you sit like that."
(J) "You're not being wise when you refuse to take your medicines."
(D) "I think you would be better off taking your medicines as your doctor prescribes."
(J) "You're not doing the right thing when you cheat on your exercises."
(D) "I think you'd feel better if you did your exercises regularly."
(J) "You have a bad temper—it's not good for you to get angry so often."
(D) "It hurts me to see you get as angry as you do."

It is worth noting that you can ask judgmental questions as well as make judgmental comments:

- "Why in the world did you do something like that?"
- "How could you possibly do that?"
- "Why don't you use the good sense God gave you?"

- "How can you possibly justify yelling at your nurse like that?"
- "Exactly what do you think you were doing when you walked around on the cold floor barefooted?"

Keep in mind that judgmental statements and questions can be harmful, and can cause friction between you and someone who is ill. Try to have a more accepting attitude, so that you will make fewer judgmental comments. The results will be well worth the effort.

6

Being Noncommittal

Abstinence from doing is often as generous as doing,
but it is not so apparent.
—MONTAIGNE

There are times when it is wise to be noncommittal when an ill person asks you questions or makes certain kinds of statements. Sometimes a definite response can do no good, and might actually be harmful. You do not need to feel obligated to respond to everything said to you. Whether it is prudent for you to respond depends on the situation, and on the possible consequences of your answer.

You may want to be noncommittal in certain types of situations:

- When you really don't know the answer to a question
- When you don't have as much information as you need to give an adequate answer to a question
- When you have an answer to a question but prefer not to give it for any of a variety of legitimate

reasons (for example, when giving it would do more harm than good)

- When you know the answer to a question that would be more appropriate to hear from someone else (for example, a doctor or nurse)
- When you don't want to answer a question until you know why the person is asking it
- When you simply want to remain neutral and not be on the spot
- When you want the person to answer his or her own question (such as when you wish to find out the person's own preference first)
- When saying nothing appears to be the best thing to do

Being noncommittal means that you avoid expressing your views, taking a position, or giving a definite answer to something an ill person says to you or asks of you. When you are noncommittal, it is important that you not appear evasive—even though you actually are evading the question. You want to communicate genuine interest, as well as a sincere desire to be responsive, lest you jeopardize your credibility with the person.

Because most politicians are skillful in the art of giving evasive answers, you may find that you can pick up many valuable pointers by studying their public comments. Try to avoid letting a sick person put you on the spot, forcing you to say something you don't really want to say.

Sometimes, making neutral comments, or saying nothing at all, is the kindest and most considerate thing you can do for a person. Your common sense, your relationship with the person, and the particulars of the specific situation all should guide you when you're deciding whether to say something or to remain silent.

Even when you choose to be noncommittal about a matter, be alert to a chance to say something to help enable the person to make the decision, or resolve the problem, on his or her own.

There are many honorable statements you can make, and questions you can ask, when you want to remain noncommittal. You will find these examples grouped into five convenient categories:

1. When asked health-related questions:

- "I'm sorry—I'm not a doctor, and I don't know enough to answer your question."
- "I'm not the right person to answer that question for you."
- "Let me discuss that with your doctor first."
- "You're be better off asking your doctor that."
- "I just don't have a clear enough view of the big picture to let me know whether you'll recover or not."
- "What do you think your nurse would say to your request?"
- "Your nurse can answer that better than I can."
- "I can't predict what's ahead—let's just take things one day at a time."

2. When you want to remain neutral:

- "I think some people would agree with you, and some wouldn't."
- "I can see two sides to the issue, and both of them have their merits."
- "You may be right—I simply don't know what is right and what is wrong in this situation."
- "I can see you feel strongly about this!"
- "Hmm . . . what you're saying is very interesting."
- "What you just said reminds me of a similar situation I heard about." (changing the subject)
- "Let's see what the pros and cons are about this."
- "You say you don't know what to do because different people are giving you different advice—hmm . . ."
- "I'm surprised to hear you say that."
- "I hear/see what you're saying."
- "Maybe so—but then again, maybe not."
- "I'm not sure about that."
- "Tell me more."
- "I really don't have anything to say about that."
- "It wouldn't be right for me to comment on that."
- "You feel as though you're being neglected, right?" (a mirroring statement)
- Remain silent, but continue to look interested.

3. When you lack the knowledge to answer:

- "I'm sorry—I don't know how to answer that."
- "I really don't know how to respond to that, and I'd rather not just guess."
- "I simply don't know—I'm sorry."
- "I'd like to answer your question but I can't—that's the $64,000 question, isn't it?"
- "I really don't know all the facts, so I'd better not try to answer that."
- "I don't know, but I'll try to find out for you."
- "I wish I had an answer for you, but I don't."
- "We don't always have answers to our questions."

4. When you want to delay your answer:

- "This is news to me—I'll need some time to think about it."
- "I don't know, but I'll do my best to find out for you."
- "Let's just wait and see."
- "What you've just told me is too important for me to answer right off the top of my head."
- "I'll need a little time to digest what you've just told me."
- "I can't give you an answer right now, but let me get back to you soon."
- Note: If you say you'll give the person an answer in the future, you are ethically obligated to do so."
- "I'll have to check on that."
- "Let's deal with that later—right now we need to . . ."

- "Let's revisit that next week."
- "I'll need to talk with the lawyer before I can answer that for you."
- "Let me pray about that, and then we can sit down and talk about it."

5. When you want the person to answer his or her own question:

- "You know better than I do what to do about that."
- "What do you think you should do?"
- "What would you like to see happen?"
- "What do you think the best solution is?"
- "You don't need me to tell you what to do."
- "Why are you asking me? You know much more about it than I do."
- "I hear you—now what?"
- "I really don't have an answer for you right now—but what do you think about it?"
- "What do you want to do about that?"
- "Why do you feel that way?"

There are all kinds of tactful noncommittal statements you can make when you want to remain neutral, when you don't know the answer, when you want to delay an answer, or when you want to enable a person to answer his or her questions. In every case, it is a good idea to take a minute to think about the best thing to say in each particular situation.

7

Being Nonresponsive

It isn't very intelligent to find answers to questions which are unanswerable.

—FONTENELLE

Generally, it is a good idea to respond to whatever an ill person has said to you. This is both the tactful and the appropriate thing to do. But there are a few occasions when it might be best to listen attentively without offering any response.

Situations in which non-responsiveness is best might include situations where:

- You are being verbally abused or insulted excessively;
- The response should come from a cleric or health professional;
- The person is benefiting from venting and you feel it advisable not to interrupt by saying anything;
- The person is complaining about a caregiver;
- You have no satisfactory answer;
- You can't fathom the strange things being said;

- You are momentarily overwhelmed by what you hear and need time to collect your thoughts;
- The person is beating up on himself or herself—for example, by saying things such as, "I don't know why I deserve to have this happen to me."
- You can't say anything helpful and your response would serve no useful purpose (and might even prove harmful);
- The person's comments are rhetorical and thus need no response, or when the ill person doesn't act as though he or she wants or expects a response.

It is wise to try to be responsive to everything an ill person says to you unless you have sound reasons for not doing so. Remember that many people consider being ignored or having their words ignored to be the supreme insult.

8

Being Silent

There is an eloquent silence.
It serves sometimes to approve, sometimes to condemn;
there is a mocking silence; there is a respectful silence.
—LA ROCHEFOUCAULD

There is a time to remain silent as well as a time to talk—and you need to be sensitive enough to know the difference. Remaining silent is difficult at times; it requires considerable patience and strong self-discipline. But when you have nothing to say, it is a good idea to say nothing.

A person's silence can be extremely meaningful. Not all silence is the same; some can say more than words do—silence can speak eloquently, and it can thunder a message. Our feelings can often best be communicated by our silence. In some situations, silence is helpful (for example, when sitting silently, holding someone who is feeling lonely) when speech would be harmful.

You should be alert for unnatural silence, because sometimes it is just as important to observe what is not said as what is said. You can learn much more about an ill person from listening to him or her than you can from talking to him or her. And prolonged silence can create tension and anxiety, which encourage a person to say something further that may be significant.

To use silence to your best advantage, keep your mouth closed while your eyes, ears, and antenna are wide open and on full alert. Silence can work to your advantage in several ways:

- Silence allows an ill person to talk freely, revealing additional valuable information.
- Silence prods the person who is speaking to say something more, to overcome the discomfort created by prolonged silence.
- Silence gives the person who is listening time to organize his or her thoughts before responding, particularly on an important matter.
- Silence gives the person who is listening time to better digest what has been said, and it gives the speaker time to rehear what he or she has just said.
- Silence enables a person to avoid saying something ill-advised.
- Silence helps the person who is listening to show the person who is speaking that he or she is taking the time to carefully consider what has been said, rather than giving an instant response to something, especially when it is important.

Because a person's silence can indicate many things, be cautious when you interpret the meaning of silence. Silence has meaning only within a certain context, so be sure to interpret the meaning of prolonged silence strictly within its specific context.

The meaning of silence can generally be interpreted in four ways:

1. Agreement with what has been said
2. Indifference to what has been said
3. Opposition to what has been said
4. An inability to respond, particularly because of a lack of energy

On the face of it, all you know when someone is silent is that he or she is not talking. Unless body language makes it unmistakable, you can't really come to any firm conclusions. When this is the case, you'll need to secure clarification, either by making a statement or by asking a question:

- "Burt, I expected some sort of response from you about what I've just said, and I'm not sure what to make of your silence."
- "Betty, I get the impression you're saying something by your silence, I can't tell what exactly—can you help me out?"

To break a lengthy silence after you've said something, try these helpful approaches:

- Lean forward toward the person, with a slight nod.
- Maintain steady eye contact, and have an expectant look on your face as you give a slight nod.
- Nod to the person, while making an open upward gesture with one hand and arm.

Remember—being ill requires a lot of energy. An ill person may be too tired or weak to talk easily, or listen alertly, particularly at certain times. Remember: there *is* such a thing as a comfortable silence. Your mere presence and availability may be all the comfort a sick person needs in many instances. Your silence communicates all that needs to be communicated at such times.

9

Being Understood

I wish he would explain his explanation.
—LORD BYRON

It is extremely difficult to be completely understood by anyone. Because of this, it is dangerous to assume that when you say something, it is understood the way you intended it to be understood. It is a mistake to assume that close, frequent contact with someone guarantees that you are going to be understood by that person. This simply is not so.

Each person is unique—different. Consequently, every person uses, and interprets, words differently. The chronically ill person's perception of things that are said and done may be quite different from that of a well person. In fact, a sick person's own perceptions of something said may vary with how he or she feels.

People tend to see and hear what is important to them, and they automatically filter out anything else. It is highly unlikely that a seriously ill person will go to the trouble of trying to view things as you view them in order to understand what you are saying or doing. If you are talking about something new or complicated, an ill person may encounter difficulty making any sense of it—in such situations, he or she may even tune you out.

The person who is speaking has the primary responsibility of making himself or herself understood. You will enhance your chances of getting understood if you get your thoughts crystal-clear in your own mind first before saying anything to anyone. It is impossible to clearly communicate to another person something that is unclear to you. (It is axiomatic that clear thinking must precede clear expression.)

It is a good idea to ask yourself these questions before saying anything important to an ill person:

1. What exactly do I want to say?
2. Why do I want to say it?
3. How can I say it most clearly?
4. Where is the best place to say it?
5. What is the best time to say it?
6. How can I make my point firmly, yet tactfully?

You promote understanding by
- Knowing what you intend to say
- Saying what you mean to say
- Meaning what you say
- Showing that you meant what you said

To be understood, you must say precisely what you intend to say. An ill person listening to you can't accurately guess what you intended to say; he or she can absorb only what you *actually* said.

You will gain better understanding if you ask yourself these four questions about the person listening to you:

1. What is his or her knowledge of the content of my message?
2. What additional information does he or she need to understand my message?
3. What is his or her attitude toward the content of my message? For example, is he or she favorable, or antagonistic?
4. How interested is he or she in the topic? For example, does he or she need to be motivated to listen?

These specific tips should help you get people to understand what you are saying:

- Create a favorable climate (e.g., comfortable and quiet).
- Say important things at the time that is best for the ill person, not the time that is most convenient for you.
- Use simple language and plain words—but don't talk down to the person.
- Be specific with what you say—don't be general or vague.
- Be direct to the point—avoid rambling.

- Tailor your words to the listener—use turn-on words, and avoid turn-off words, when speaking to an ill person.
- Say important things more than once, and say them in different ways.
- Emphasize important points you are making by saying, "This is important for you to understand if you want to sleep better" or "Let me be clear about this because it is important to your recovery program."
- Tell the person what you are going to say, then say it to him or her, then tell him or her what you have said.
- Use clear, definite transitions when leaving one point and moving on to the next one: "Now I want to move on to another idea about how you can sleep better."
- Send a consistent message—avoid using ambiguous words that can be interpreted several ways. Also, make sure that your words, voice, and body language all say the same thing. And be certain that you are telling the ill person the same things that other people are telling him or her on important matters (e.g., his or her health condition).
- Be brief. Limit the amount of content that you share at any one time. (Don't overwhelm him or her with information, lest you confuse him or her, causing him or her to tune out.)
- Refrain from mixing unimportant information with important information.

As stated previously, it is a big mistake to simply assume that you have been understood when you've said something. You can just as easily be misunderstood as understood.

The only way to verify that you have been understood is to obtain feedback. These proven techniques can help you secure the necessary feedback:

- Ask the person to repeat the essence of what you said in his or her own words: "What is your understanding of what I've just said?"
- Ask for specific reactions: "What do you think about my suggestions for helping you sleep better?"
- Ask for any anticipated problems: "If you were to change your bedtime, what problems would it cause?"
- Ask the person if he or she has any questions: "I've said quite a lot about your sleeping, so I expect you probably have some questions; what are they?" Refrain from saying, "Do you understand what I've said?" This encourages an affirmative reply whether or not the person has understood you.
- While you are talking, watch intently for any body language clues that might indicate that the person is confused (e.g., blank facial expressions, squirming, looking around).

You can gain confirmation that you have been understood even if the ill person is unable to speak; for example, you could ask him or her to blink once for a yes response and repeatedly for a no answer. Or, assuming the person can move his or her hands, you could ask him or her to squeeze your hand once for a yes response and twice for a no response.

It may help you to appreciate the difficulty of getting understood if you keep this quotation in mind: "I know you believe you understand what you think I've said, but I am sure you realize that what you heard is not what I meant."

10

Disagreeing

Disputation cannot be held without reprehension.
—MONTAIGNE

Some disagreement is inevitable among human beings, since we are all unique, all different. We have different thoughts, feelings, beliefs, values, and opinions, so it follows that some disagreement between you and someone who is ill is natural, and in fact to be expected.

You and the person for whom you are caring are entitled to have, and to air, different viewpoints. It is okay to be open about the fact you disagree on important matters. But on minor points of disagreement you may want to remain silent, refraining from expressing your disagreement. Why risk creating tension by disagreeing over something trivial?

And although it is okay to disagree, it is not okay to be nasty, or to take every disagreement personally. If you feel you are being verbally attacked, control your emotions; realize that the attack is on your thoughts or ideas, and not on you as a person.

Whenever you and an ill person disagree, try to do so agreeably. Do your best to agree in principle, if possible—even though you disagree on the details of a matter. Emphasize your points of agreement and downplay your areas of disagreement. Try to gain agreement on your sources of disagreement, and then agree to disagree on these points if necessary. Sometimes the term *difference of opinion* is preferable to *disagreement*, being simply a less emotionally charged way of saying the same thing.

It is important to know three things when disagreeing with an ill person:

1. Know when, and when not, to press a point; for example, it is unwise to press a point when the other person is tired, hungry, irritable, or in pain.

2. Know which matters can, and can't, be disputed. Know the person's blind spots, prejudices, and hot buttons. Know when his or her convictions are so strong that he or she can't discuss them objectively.

3. Know how to disagree without being disagreeable. By making carefully worded, inoffensive statements, you can minimize the chances of evoking strong antagonistic reactions. If you press a point hard and vigorously, you can expect a stronger, more vigorous reaction than if you had explained your position in a low-key, conversational manner.

Never quarrel! No one wins a fight. Quarreling creates more heat than light. And refrain from talking loudly, too—no one wins a shouting match, either. Strive to state your views tactfully, in order to avoid wounding fragile egos. If your manner makes a person feel defensive, you will cause the person to become close-minded. Do your best to always give the ill person an easy out; never put him or her in a corner with no escape. Instead, try to find a way for him or her to save face, and to maintain his or her self-esteem.

Listen intently to the other person's point of view and the reasons for it (and realize that the other person thinks that he or she is just as right as you believe you are). Listen without interrupting with your counterpoints, and pause before you do say anything. If you respond immediately, it suggests to the other person that you haven't really listened to him or her or considered what he or she said.

Whenever you respond, do so briefly. Get directly to the point, and clearly explain the reasons for your viewpoint. It is a mistake to overwhelm the ill person by presenting too many counterpoints. If you say too much, the other person may simply stop listening and tune you out entirely.

Choosing the best way to disagree depends on four factors:

1. The importance of the issue being discussed
2. The intensity of the person's feelings about the topic
3. The degree of compatibility between the two parties
4. The closeness of the relationship (e.g., fellow worker, family member)

Some disagreements are highly charged emotionally, and can be so strong and bitter that they can do lasting harm to your relationship. Since your goal is to help the ill person, don't risk creating animosity by disagreeing in the wrong way.

You can minimize causing resentment when disagreeing if you make statements or ask questions in a diplomatic manner.

Recommended Statements

- "We don't seem to be moving ahead with our discussion, so why don't we delay a decision until we can both give the matter more thought?"
- "Most of what you say makes sense to me, and you could be right—but I wonder if this idea might also make sense."
- "I can go along with much of what you are saying, but I'd like to make a suggestion for you to consider."
- "As you know, we agree on most things, but I differ with you somewhat on this matter, and I wonder if you'd be willing to reconsider."
- "We know what we disagree on, but now let's see what we agree on."
- "I think that with some give and take from both of us, we can come to an agreement together."
- "I've listened carefully to all you've said, and I'd like for you to listen to me now—fair enough?"

- "You've given me something new to think about—now let me give you something new to consider."

Recommended Questions
- "What do you think a fair solution would be?"
- "How would you like to see our differences resolved?"
- "How can I help you with the problem in a way that is acceptable to you?"
- "What are we able to agree on?"
- "How do you think we should proceed, since we see this matter differently?"
- "What do you think would happen if we were to do this?"

In the final analysis, it is important to know what is worth agreeing and disagreeing over, and how to reconcile differences in a mutually acceptable manner.

11

Discussing Dreams

A dream that is not understood is like
a letter that is not opened.
—The Talmud

People's dreams can be significant, especially the dreams of the critically ill. Dreams often spring from strong emotions and contain clues about the concerns, needs, and fears of the person dreaming. Dreams can be both comforting and frightening, and can be especially meaningful when the person dreaming is close to death.

When a person dreams, his or her unconscious mind brings thoughts and feelings to the attention of the conscious self. Through this process, the person becomes aware of things that were previously unknown and hidden from his or her conscious mind.

Dreams appear to have three primary functions for those who are dying:

1. They help those who are dying come to grips with their fears and anxieties.
2. They help reconcile alienated relatives.

3. They help those who are dying discover the real
   meaning of their lives.

Despite years of intense study by psychiatrists and
clinical psychologists, dreams remain largely a mystery;
more remains unknown about dreams than is known. But
there is no doubt that dreams are highly significant. We do
know that the most important dreams are those that are
the most vivid, as well as those that are recurring and that
are dreamed in a progressive series.

The accurate interpretation of dreams is difficult, if not
impossible. Even renowned psychiatrist Sigmund Freud,
still acknowledged as the leading authority on dream
analysis, frequently encountered difficulty interpreting
dreams. Do not try to interpret anyone's dreams. The best
person to interpret the meaning of a sick person's dreams
is the sick person.

By listening carefully to a person relate his or her
dreams, you can help him or her explore the thoughts and
feelings revealed by the dreams. By asking for details about
dreams, you encourage an ill person to discuss the needs
and fears the dreams suggest. For example, you can ask
questions such as the following:

- "What do you think the dream is saying?"
- "What feelings do you have about the dream?"
- "Have you had this dream before?"
- "How often have you had this dream?"
- "Are you having this dream more frequently?"

If the dream involved feelings of loneliness and isolation, you can discuss these feelings to learn why the person feels that way, and what he or she thinks can be done to overcome these feelings. Many times merely relating a dream helps the dreamer solve the problem associated with it. A nightmare, for example, can be a warning about some unresolved issue. The dream focuses on the problem and helps resolve it.

Be sure to let the person who had the dream do most of the talking. Your role is to listen patiently, and with interest, and to ask occasional leading questions to aid the thinking of the dreamer. Your role is not to try, in any way, to interpret the dream for the person.

An analysis of the dreams of those who are dying suggests that three kinds of dreams occur repeatedly under such circumstances:

1. Seeing and talking with people who have died—usually family members.
2. Finding a type of freedom by flying about, perhaps like a bird or a weather balloon.
3. Beginning some kind of journey.

Although many uncertainties surround the meaning of people's dreams, one thing is certain: it is a serious mistake to ignore or discount the dreams of those who are critically ill.

12

Giving and Receiving Criticism

People ask you for criticism, but they only want praise.
—W. Somerset Maugham

Giving Criticism

There are times when you need to criticize ill people for their own good. They are entitled to be leveled with about problems that they are causing; you can't just pretend there are no problems when problems actually exist. Simply ignoring problems doesn't make sense— they need to be dealt with, no matter how reluctant you are to do so. So criticize when it is necessary—but do it in the proper way.

Be careful when criticizing a sick person; no one likes to be criticized, especially people who may be feeling sick and depressed. In fact, oddly enough, people frequently resent being criticized even when they have requested criticism from you.

It is a good idea to ask yourself these questions before criticizing an ill person:

- What is my specific purpose? What do I want to achieve with my criticism?
- What reactions do I predict? Will the criticism be helpful, or harmful? Could it make matters even worse?
- Is my criticism fair and reasonable?
- What exactly do I need to say? How can I best say it?
- What is the best time, and the best place, to do it?
- How can I minimize resistance to, and enhance receptivity of, my criticism?

The following recommendations for criticizing people should help answer the preceding questions, and should serve to make your criticizing more effective:

- Offer all criticism in a friendly, helpful, and kindly manner.
- Be calm, avoiding any hint of anger or irritation.
- Assure the person that your criticism is meant to be helpful and constructive.
- Emphasize the future improvement sought, rather than fault-finding with past or current behavior: "If you eat your meals regularly, you'll feel stronger, rest better, and be more energetic."
- Criticize only specific attitudes and behavior: "Your refusal to bathe is causing hygienic problems that concern your nurse. You need to bathe regularly to be clean and feel better."

- Say what needs to be said in a way that protects the person's feelings: "I know you were feeling tired and in pain when you refused to cooperate with your physical therapist, but you need to engage in physical therapy faithfully so that you can improve your strength. How can we make therapy less objectionable to you?"
- Watch your tone of voice while criticizing: keep it pleasant and low-pitched; avoid any sarcasm or ridicule.
- Use simple, clear, easily understood language.
- State your criticism as tactfully as you can, but don't be so diplomatic and indirect that the person misses the point you are making.
- Refrain from giving any commands or making any demands: "You need to take physical therapy regularly and cooperate fully with your physical therapist—no ifs, ands, or buts about it."
- Pick the best time of day for sharing your criticism. This is usually early in the day, while the person is feeling fresh, rather than at the end of the day, when he or she is more likely to feel tired and irritable.
- Make certain that your words, tone of voice, and body language all send the same message. Avoid sending mixed signals at all cost.
- Use *I* statements rather than *you* statements. Own your criticism, and take responsibility for it: "I notice that you have stopped taking your medicine.

This bothers me, because you need to take your pills, so that you will feel more comfortable and sleep better."

- Describe the problem rather than making judgments about it: "Jim, you haven't been taking your pain pills for three days now, and yet you are complaining that you are constantly in pain—don't you think you should resume taking them?"

Receiving Criticism

Chronically ill people are frequently quite critical about people and events. They have their own criticisms and complaints about how others are treating them; this is natural and to be expected.

A chronically ill friend or family member may criticize you about almost anything. It is very hard to accept such criticism graciously when you have been doing your best, and making personal sacrifices, to try to help the person. In fact, it is natural for you to become somewhat defensive, and to resent being criticized in such an instance.

Remember, the mark of a secure, well-adjusted person is his or her ability to accept criticism graciously and gracefully.

Be open-minded when you are being criticized. The criticism may be deserved, and what it reveals may help you care for the ill person better. Try to understand not only the criticism, but also why the person is giving it; try to detect the motive behind it. For example, the person may need to let off steam after reaching the boiling point with his or her nurse's increasing demands, and you may simply have been the next person he or she saw—so you become his or her punching bag for whatever gripes come to mind.

In such a situation, try not to take the attack personally, or to become defensive and hostile in return. Be willing to control your emotions, and to hear the person out.

You will find certain kinds of responses particularly effective when you are being criticized:

- "Hmm—I didn't realize I did that. Will you tell me more about it so I get a better idea of what I do?"
- "I appreciate your candor, but I'm a little unclear on a couple of things you said; could you give me some examples of what I've done that you especially object to?"
- "I'm concerned that you feel I've been neglecting you—I wasn't aware you felt this way."
- "I'm sorry you feel that way—I'll work to do better in the future."

Neither criticizing nor being criticized is pleasant, but both can be beneficial when the goal is to be helpful, and when they are done in the right way.

13

Giving and Receiving Feedback

*Men no longer test words to see what the truth is in them;
the majority are only interested in knowing
what their effect will be.*
—Theodor Haecker

The potential for feedback is present in all conversations; the problem is how to give it, and how to get it. Feedback is too important to leave to happenstance. Effective feedback requires a deliberate effort. And it is particularly important that ill people give and receive feedback.

Feedback completes the communication cycle. It is the reaction or response of the listener to what the person who is speaking has said. Feedback is the only way you have of verifying that you understand something that was said to you, and the only way for you to confirm that something you have said is understood by the person who is listening to you. It is foolhardy to simply assume that you understand or are understood. Feedback is a reciprocal process that involves the exchanging of feelings, facts, and ideas.

Effective feedback requires that the person speaking be honest and candid with his or her message, and that the person listening be willing to receive it. It also requires that the person speaking and the person listening trust each other. In addition, both parties must be open to feedback, and must view the feedback as being given with helpful, rather than harmful, intent.

The speaker's and listener's perceived attitudes have a significant effect on both the type and extent of feedback. For example, people are less inclined to share honest feedback regularly if they don't think the receiver is receptive to the message and will not appreciate the effort expended in providing it. Also, try to minimize the use of *me* and *my*.

Giving Feedback

It is important to avoid giving feedback that is threatening to an ill individual, because doing so is likely to make him or her defensive. And the more defensive the person listening becomes, the less likely it is that he or she will be able to hear what you have actually said, and to understand what you really mean. Before giving feedback, know what your specific purpose is. Say what you need to say in a low-key, tactful manner of the sort that you think will be most favorably received by the person you're addressing.

The best feedback is specific, rather than general. For example, when discussing a sick person's progress in building up leg strength, it is better to say, "If you do your leg exercise faithfully, you will improve your legs' strength and will be able to walk sooner," than to say, "You need to improve your exercises to feel better."

Time your feedback for optimal results. Generally, prompt feedback is preferable to delayed feedback. Furthermore, try to time your feedback at the best time for the ill person, even if it is not the most convenient time for you. Feedback given at a bad time can be significantly less helpful, and sometimes even harmful— for example, well-intended and much-needed feedback may be rejected by someone who is preoccupied or in pain. Additionally, helpful feedback may be taken the wrong way, even resented, if the ill person is especially tired or is in a bad mood.

Think first before providing feedback—especially highly important feedback. Consider the possible consequences ahead of time, and try to predict the person's reactions. Show your compassion by tailoring the wording of the feedback to the particular person. Use plain, simple language, and refrain from using ambiguous words or fancy language with which the ill person may be unfamiliar. The easier your feedback is to understand, the better.

Limit the amount of feedback you dispense to what the sick individual can absorb at a sitting, rather than the entirety of the feedback you have ready to give; don't overload the person with excessive information. (When you overload an ill person with too much feedback, you automatically reduce its effectiveness.) Any time you give a person more information than he or she can digest, you are meeting your needs rather than his or hers. Remember—you want to have your feedback viewed as being helpful instead of as an unwelcome imposition.

Here are some additional tips for giving feedback:

- Make it clear to the person that the feedback is meant to be positive and helpful.
- Make sure the receiver is paying attention, and is in a mood to listen.
- Give feedback when the matter is fresh in both your minds.
- Be humble—avoid communicating that you think that you know more than the other person.
- Furnish feedback calmly and in a low-key manner.
- Provide both positive and negative feedback.
- Separate the actual facts from your own perceptions.
- Include only important information.
- Allow plenty of time—never rush it.
- Be descriptive, not judgmental. For example, say, "You took your medicine only once yesterday instead of the prescribed four times," rather than, "You are wrong not to take your medicine as prescribed by your doctor."
- Bear in mind—your goal is to have your feedback understood, believed, and accepted.
- Verify that the person understands your feedback by asking the person to restate what you've said in his or her own words.

Receiving Feedback

Now, let's examine several ideas for you to secure feedback from an ill person:

- Begin by recognizing the importance of such feedback.
- Assure the person that you welcome and appreciate feedback, and in no way resent it.
- Ask for feedback in a polite, respectful way, without demanding it.
- Explain how the person will benefit from giving you feedback; for example, "If you tell me what you want to eat, I'll be able to cook it for you."
- Show great interest in what the person is telling you.
- Pay attention not only to the person's words when offering feedback, but also to his or her body language while doing so.
- Ask general (open-ended) questions first, followed by specific probing questions to secure more information.
- Use silence, and lean toward the person with an expectant look to encourage him or her to respond.
- Verify you understand what you've been told.
- Thank the person for his or her assistance, expressing your sincere appreciation.

Remember: giving and getting essential feedback is a necessity—not a luxury.

14

Giving and Receiving Praise

*The deepest principle of human nature is
the craving to be appreciated.*
—William James

All people like to be praised and appreciated; Mark Twain emphasized the importance of praise by saying, "I can live for two months on a good compliment." In particular, ill people need to feel valued.

Look for opportunities to offer genuine praise to an ill person. When he or she does something well, don't hesitate to say so. For example, you might say, "Your nurse tells me that you have increased your strength-building exercises by 10 percent—this is great news, and I'm proud of you." But be sure to be honest—give compliments only when they are truly deserved, or they will ring hollow.

Giving Praise

You should know how to praise an ill person so that it really counts. Your praise will have the greatest impact if you apply the following principles:

- Be specific about what you're praising; for example, "I think you really look nice today—and I especially like your colorful blouse."
- Be enthusiastic, and act like you enjoy complimenting the person.
- Be spontaneous—unsolicited praise comes across as the most sincere.
- Adapt your praise to the person's personality. For example, if the person is quiet and modest, make your praise more indirect: "I wonder, since you have such a good eye for color, if you would tell me what color you think I should paint the kitchen."
- Do it promptly—if you wait too long to compliment someone or something, your compliment loses its value.
- Select the most appropriate time and place to compliment the person. Many times it is best to praise a person privately, so you don't risk embarrassing him or her in front of others.
- Act comfortable, and take your time complimenting—never rush your compliment.
- Share compliments you've heard others pay the person secondhand; for example, "Several of the family have remarked on how much better you are walking the past few days."

Just as there are wise things to do when complimenting a sick individual, there are unwise things to do. If done improperly, your attempt to be positive by giving praise can harm your shared relationship.

Try to avoid making certain types of mistakes when praising an ill person:

- Don't act superior, condescending, or patronizing when offering a compliment; for example, "Good for you—I was wondering when you'd see the light and change doctors."
- Don't praise in an effort to manipulate. This kind of praise is transparent, and creates suspicion and resentment.
- Don't flatter the person by heaping excessive compliments. Gushing praise appears insincere and can make the person feel embarrassed—and make them doubt your motives.
- Don't act uncomfortable or embarrassed while paying a compliment; this will make the recipient feel uncomfortable.
- Don't rush a compliment as if you can't wait to get it over with.
- Don't pay a compliment sarcastically or in order to ridicule the person; for example, "I'm glad to see you're finally getting out of bed and doing your exercises like you are supposed to."

Receiving Praise

Praise is not a one-way street. On occasion, an ill person will compliment you for being so caring and helpful. It is important that you accept such compliments graciously, and without acting uncomfortable or embarrassed.

Certain responses are actually put-downs and insults, and should be avoided:

- "Don't thank me—I didn't really do anything much."
- "Oh, stop it! I don't deserve any praise for the little bit I've done."
- "I was beginning to wonder if you were ever going to notice all the hard work I put into the garden."

Instead of such ill-advised comments, make brief, effective responses of a different sort:

- "Thank you."
- "Thank you—I was happy to be able to help."
- "Thanks for mentioning it—I was hoping the new menu would be more appetizing."
- "I really appreciate your kind words."

Such short but sincere replies are very effective when acknowledging your appreciation at being complimented. Such kinds of responses are always appropriate and contain nothing that might offend the person who has complimented you.

15

Asking Questions

He who asks a question is a fool for five minutes; he who does not ask a question remains a fool forever.
—Chinese Proverb

There are various questions you can ask an ill person that could be helpful. To be helpful, a question needs to
- Be properly worded
- Be said in the right way
- Be asked at the best time

For convenience and easy reference, the following list of helpful questions has been organized into five categories:

1. Offering help and comfort:
- "How can I make you feel more comfortable?"
- "How can I help you today?"
- "Would you like any company?"
- "Is there anything I can do for you right now?"
- "How can I help you most?"
- "Would it be helpful if I were to . . . ?"

- "What do you need today?"
- "How can I help you deal with your boredom?"
- "Are you getting the help you need?"

2. Encouraging conversation:

- "Why do you say that?"
- "What do you have to say about . . . ?"
- "Do you want to say anything more about that?"
- "What would you like to talk about now?"
- "What are your thoughts about . . . ?"
- "Did I hear you correctly when you said . . . ?"
- "How do you feel about . . . ?"
- "What's on your mind today?"
- "What is your opinion of . . . ?"
- "Which of your achievements are you proudest of?"
- "How are your children doing these days?"

3. Learning about their daily living:

- "What's happening in your life?"
- "What makes your days go better?"
- "What do you intend to do today that interests you?"
- "Is there anything you would like to do together?"
- "What would you like to do today?"
- "How is your family doing?"
- "How would you like to live the rest of your life?"

4. Discussing health condition:

- "Well, how are you feeling today?"
- "How are things going?"
- "What's going on regarding your back pain?"
- "What do you mean when you say you are hurting?"
- "What feelings do you have about your new diagnosis?"
- "Are there any health problems you would like to discuss with me?"
- "Can you help me understand how you are doing?"
- "Would you tell me when the pain began, and what you think caused it?"
- "On a scale of 1–10, how is your pain today?"

5. Sharing concerns and anxieties:

- "What troubles you about your health insurance?"
- "Are there any problems you want to discuss with me today?"
- "Do you want to talk about God with me today, or do you want me to read some scripture?"
- "Are any family issues still bothering you that you want to discuss further?"
- "What is your plan for dealing with your family's resentment over your condition?"
- "Are you still concerned about . . . ?"
- "Are you feeling less anxious about . . . ?"

Clearly, there is an infinite number of questions you could ask, and topics you could discuss, to attempt to help a chronically ill person feel better. The most important point is that your questions need to deal with matters that are relevant to the well-being of the ailing individual. Always strive to make your questions be helpful, and never harmful.

16

Types of Questions to Ask

Ask, and it shall be given you, seek and ye shall find.
—Matthew 7:7

You need to ask questions to gain insights into the thoughts and feelings of someone who is ill. The right questions need to be asked in the right way. You can't get good answers from bad questions; the quality of an answer is directly related to the quality of the questions. Thus, you need to carefully consider the intent and wording of a question before you ask it.

An effective question is

- Clear and free of ambiguity
- Concise and directly to the point
- Simply stated in plain language
- Nonjudgmental
- Free of clues about the preferred answer
- Relevant, getting to the crux of the matter
- Worded in such a way that it makes giving an evasive answer difficult

- Free of intimidation, avoiding putting the person questioned on the defensive
- Nonintrusive, respecting a person's need for privacy

The two major purposes for asking questions are to clarify what was said and to learn more about what was said, but there are several other worthwhile reasons for asking questions:

- Stalling for time so you can consider a question you've been asked before responding to it
- Avoiding answering a question you don't want to answer
- Learning the intent or reasons behind a question
- Leading a questioner to think of something new, or changing the direction of the conversation

There are two kinds of questions—general and specific. A general question sets no boundaries on the person's answer, whereas a specific question limits the parameters of the response. These examples will assist you to understand the differences between general (G) and specific (S) questions:

- (G) "What do you think about the new physical therapist?"
- (S) "How do you think the new physical therapist's type of massage will help you?"
- (G) "How do you feel today?"
- (S) "How does your back feel today?"

Ask general questions to encourage the ill person to say anything he or she wants to. Conversely, ask specific, narrow questions to encourage the person to give a more restricted answer to your questions.

In addition to classifying questions as general and specific, questions can be categorized as open- and close-ended.

In most situations, open-ended questions are preferable to close-ended if you want to probe without giving any clues as to what you are thinking or wanting to hear. Ask open-ended questions if you want to force the person to provide details rather than respond only with a yes or no (which is possible with close-ended questions). Open-ended questions also are best for allowing the person to air the concerns foremost in his or her mind.

Open-ended questions frequently start with the words how and why, and sometimes what, could, and would, which tend to generate longer answers. On the other hand, close-ended questions often begin with the words did, is, or, are, can, and will. These kinds of questions can be answered with a simple yes or no, without any elaboration.

Here are a few examples of open- (O) and closed- (C) ended questions:

(O) "How have you been sleeping?"
(C) "Have you been sleeping well?"
(O) "How do you like your new doctor?"
(C) "Do you like your new doctor?"
(O) "Why do you think your medicine is helping you?"
(C) "Is your new medicine helping you?"

Whatever type of question you elect to use, try to reduce the ill person's apprehension, and make him or her feel less threatened, by explaining the reason for your question before you ask it. For example, "You keep saying you don't like physical therapy; would you like to change physical therapists?"

You will also reduce the person's defensiveness if you ask all your questions in a conversational style and make them sound as spontaneous as possible. Try not to come across as a detective pressing a subject for a confession. Since you are not an interrogator, make sure you don't sound like one.

It is best to ask only one question at a time, in order to give the person time to think about his or her answer. If the ill person is unduly hesitant or is having trouble answering, you can say, "Excuse me—let me ask the question another way." By rephrasing the question, you may be able to make it more precise and clearer for the person you are questioning. Also, whenever a person is slow in answering something, resist the temptation to jump in to help the person answer it—or, worse yet, to answer your own question.

If you suspect that the sick person is trying to word his or her answer in an evasive manner or is holding something back, it is a good idea to later ask the same question in a different way to gain further insights. And whenever the person answers a question, be certain that you understand the answer before you ask another question.

To get truthful responses to your questions, word all your questions in neutral language; this will prevent your offering any clues as to the answer you desire. Try not to use slanted wording, or to provide any clues by your body language. For example, your face should show neither approval or disapproval while the person is answering any of your questions. Look interested—but not judgmental.

It is a mistake to ask leading or loaded questions:

- "Don't you think it is time for you to resume your exercises?"
- "Don't you agree that you should follow your doctor's instructions more faithfully?"
- "I think you should get more sleep—what do you think?"

Try not to ask too many *why* questions, because they tend to put the person on the spot by pressuring him or her to justify his or her responses. Whenever possible, substitute *how* or *what* questions. For example, instead of asking, "Why do you refuse to eat your meals?" ask "What can I do to help you want to eat your meals?" or "How can I get you to eat your meals?"

Remember that asking questions is expected, necessary, and appropriate when you are dealing with sick people. The only dumb question is the unasked one—so feel free to ask any questions that you believe are in the ill person's best interests.

17

Saying No

I like the saying of no better than the saying of yes.
—Ralph Waldo Emerson

Chronically ill people, despite their desire not to be a burden on people, do need to request that you do things for them from time to time. This is only natural—it is to be expected. But much as you would like to say yes to all such requests, you can't always. Saying yes all the time is not a realistic expectation; sometimes there is simply no way you can meet some requests, regardless of how legitimate they are. You are only one person with many demands on your time and energy. You can't be—and can't expect to be—all things to all people at all times. It's simply impossible.

A responsible no, based on sound reasons and the particular circumstances, is sometimes preferable to giving an irresponsible yes response just to be nice and agreeable. And sometimes saying no to a request is not only necessary, but in the ill person's best interests—for example, when an ill person requests a food that is forbidden by the doctor.

You shouldn't feel guilt over denying an unwise request, or one that it is impossible for you to honor. You are acting in an honorable manner when you say no to certain requests.

Granted—saying no to a friend's or family member's request is hard, and may even be extremely unpleasant. And fairness dictates that when you say no to a request, you always base your refusal on sound reasons, and explain them to the ill person, clearly, patiently, and kindly. Saying no simply requires that you have the courage to be what you should be, and to do what you believe to be right when dealing with a chronically ill person.

Fortunately, it is possible to say no in such a loving, gracious manner that your refusal is accepted in an equally gracious manner. Here are a few things that have proven effective in many instances:

- Listen attentively, and show genuine interest in what the person is requesting.
- Try your best to understand not only the request itself but why it is being made. For example, the person may be tired of eating the same bland food, and thus may be requesting some spicy food simply for variety.
- Repeat the request to ensure that you understand it, and to show the requesting party that you do understand it.
- Take time to consider the request, to demonstrate to the person that you are giving the request careful

thought (avoid giving the impression that you are denying the request arbitrarily, without even thinking it over). You must be fair and reasonable—take pains to show that you are.

- Explain clearly and patiently, in a conversational tone, the reasons why you must deny the request. For example, "I understand that eating the same bland food gets old, but as you know, spicy foods upset your stomach and interfere with your sleep."
- Say no politely but decisively—gently, but with conviction.
- Be sure to show compassion with your tone of voice, your choice of words, and your facial expressions.
- If possible, think of another way to meet the need the request represents. If you can identify a way to do so, offer it as a low-key suggestion. For example, "Suppose we try to broaden the menu, and to prepare it somewhat differently."

As stated earlier, saying no to certain requests may be the best way of showing that you sincerely care for a person, and that you are willing to put his or her well-being above all other considerations. The ill person may not like your denial of his or her requests at the moment, but in the long run, he or she will respect you for doing what is right.

18

Saying the Right Thing

The important thing about any word
is how you understand it.
—Publilius Syrus

Words have inexact meaning. Words are always an approximation, much as a map is an approximation of the actual territory depicted. The meaning of words is always contextual. Meaning is in people—not in the words themselves. The meaning of words is intensely personal; the same words have different meanings to different people.

Since words have no meaning in and of themselves, you must do your best to select the words that most precisely say what you actually mean to say. Even a slight difference in words used can cause tremendous differences in the way they are interpreted. As Mark Twain said, "The difference between the right word and the almost right word is the difference between lightning and the lightning bug." Take a look at the difference between positive words, such as determination, zeal, and conviction, and their negative counterparts stubbornness, fanaticism, and bias.

Think before choosing the words you use when saying anything important to a sick person. Ask yourself these questions to guide you in selecting the best words to use:

- What exactly do I want to say?
- How can I best say what I want to say?
- How is the person I'm talking with likely to react to what I have to say?

Your goal is to choose words that are as clear and un-ambiguous as possible. In order to gain understanding and acceptance for what you have to say, say what you really intend to say, say it like you mean it—and show that you mean it. You want your words to be understood exactly as you intended them to be understood.

Recognize the tremendous power of words, which have the power to arouse every human emotion. Note the strong emotions associated with these phrases:

- "Damn the torpedoes—full speed ahead!"
- "Remember the Alamo!"
- "I regret that I have but one life to give for my country."
- "As for me, give me liberty or death."
- "I hate you."/"I love you."
- "He is a pervert."/"He is a child molester."
- "She is a liberal."/"She is a conservative."

Thus, it is wise to constantly think of the power of words when dealing with an ill person. Your words can help heal a person, or can make him or her feel worse; they can inspire, or demoralize, an ailing person. Your words can make your visits welcomed, or dreaded.

To improve your use of words, keep these points firmly in mind:

- Get what you want to say clear in your own mind before you say anything.
- Adapt your vocabulary level to the ill person's ability to comprehend words.
- Use words that are known and familiar to the person listening.
- Choose words that are viewed favorably by the other person. For example, if the person is a strong conservative politically, it would be smart to avoid statements such as, "You have a liberal opportunity to exercise," or to refrain from talking about the person doing certain things for his or her own welfare—use *benefit* instead.
- Express yourself plainly and simply. Use short words, and avoid long sentences. Remember that the truly big person uses small words.
- State things briefly, and get directly to the point— avoid rambling and the giving of excessive details.
- Emphasize the key points you are making, and explain important things a couple of times using different words.
- Pause after important points to let them sink in.
- Be specific: use concrete words, rather than speaking

in generalities and abstractions—remember that sloppy language causes sloppy understanding.

- Offer examples and anecdotes related to the person's experience to help make clear what you are saying.
- Use precise, unambiguous words that say exactly what you want to say—avoid nuances and subtlety.
- Select socially acceptable, tactful words—avoid profanity and harsh speech.
- Decide on the best order in which to present your ideas. For example, does the person with whom you are talking prefer conclusions followed by background information, or background information followed by conclusions?
- Decide whether it is preferable to let the person draw his or her own conclusions from what you've said, or for you to help the person form his or her conclusions.
- Speak at sufficient volume. Pronounce your words distinctly, and refrain from muttering.
- Use picture words to create mental images to promote understanding: "the little red schoolhouse."
- Use words that are compatible with the way the ill person thinks, by using words that match the person's preferred way of thinking. If you do this, he or she will feel more comfortable with you and understand you better. For example, some people use primarily visual words, whereas others use auditory words—still others use tactile words. Look for these

verbal clues to discover the person's preferred way of thinking, and then adjust your wording based on these preferences.

Verbal Clues as to Preferences	**Responses Related to Verbal Clues**
1. Give me the big picture.	1. Here's how it looks to me.
2. That doesn't sound right to me.	2. Please listen to my reasons.
3. I don't have a feel for what you are telling me yet.	3. Let me touch base with you later, after I've had a chance to think about it.

Try to say things in as soothing, noninflammatory a manner as possible. To do this avoid saying these inflammatory or red flag words:

- You should
- Don't you remember anything I tell you
- You ought
- As I keep telling you
- I told you so
- As I told you many times before
- This is the way it is—period
- You aren't able to do that
- I know what is best for you
- Why can't you ever cooperate?

- I don't know why you find it so hard to understand such a simple request

Although your words are important, there is no magic formula for their proper use. Nor is there a magic formula for knowing what to say to all chronically ill people in all situations. All you can do is rely on your best judgment, and play it by ear.

In the final analysis, what you say and how you say it may be important, but the thing that counts the most is your being present—just being with the chronically ill person.

19

Sharing Bad News

Though it be honest, it is never good to bring bad news.
—WILLIAM SHAKESPEARE

None of us likes to convey bad news to anyone. This is especially true when the recipient of the news is enduring the hardships that accompany being chronically ill; we feel that such a person has things bad enough just being seriously ill.

We tend to feel inadequate, reluctant, and anxious when we need to give bad news to anyone. Sometimes we may even feel somewhat guilty, because we know that receiving bad news upsets people, and we don't like to upset anyone. We also fear being the messenger of sad tidings, because we know that messengers are frequently blamed for their bad news—unfair as this is.

Nevertheless, people—and remember, the sick are still people—are entitled to hear the truth about things; you have the ethical obligation to present bad news, and to do it truthfully. Experience indicates that most people want to know the truth concerning bad news. And if you take the right precautions when sharing bad news, it doesn't usually damage your relationship with the person. Concentrate on how to most sensitively and helpfully share the bad news, rather than on whether or not you should.

Consider two things in particular when deciding how to share bad news:

1. Consider how to best divulge it—how to tailor your approach to the individual's personality and to the situation.
2. Consider how to listen and respond effectively—how to show compassion and empathy about the emotions expressed.

The manner in which you share the truth is crucial. Having the right attitude is the key to sharing bad news effectively. You must balance the need to be candid with the need to soften the blow in order to protect the sick person's state of mind. Sharing bad news calls for heart-to-heart and gut-to-gut—rather than mind-to-mind—communication. And *sharing* bad news is preferable to merely delivering it—an important distinction.

Your approach to sharing bad news, and the manner in which you actually share the news, helps determine how favorably bad news is received:

- Show your concern and compassion for the person in both your words and your actions.
- Choose the best time to share the news (don't wait too long).

- Select a quiet, private place.
- Sit down near the person.
- Get straight to the point, but without being abrupt.
- State the basic facts objectively, briefly, and simply (for now, leave out any unnecessary details).
- Talk calmly, in a soothing, reassuring tone of voice.
- Speak distinctly and avoid rushing your words.
- Allow the person to express anger and grief after hearing the bad news—let him or her cry without interfering.
- Listen patiently to the person—hear him or her out.
- Offer, sincerely, to help. Be sure to say, "What can I do to help you?" or, "How can I help you?" rather than, "Let me know if I can help you."
- Make it clear you are available, that you are "there," for the person—not only now, but later as well.
- At a later time, repeat your offer to help if the person declined it initially.

Keep your attention on the ill person's feelings the entire time, even though you may be experiencing intense feelings yourself. Be sure to avoid trite and meaningless comments such as

- "I'm sorry to have to tell you this."
- "I know exactly how you feel."
- "The same thing happened to me."
- "Be brave—you're strong enough to overcome this."
- "Now, here is what I'd do if I were you . . ."

- "This is awful, but remember—we grow from tragedies like these."
- "This will make you a stronger person."
- "It's God's will."

As disagreeable as sharing bad news may be, it is sometimes necessary. Bad news doesn't simply disappear if we ignore it.

It is also wise to spend some time considering who might be the best person to share a particular piece of bad news. You may be, or perhaps someone else may be. And consider, too, whether it might be best to have several loved ones present when the bad news is shared; the best interests of the ill person should be the determining factor when you make this decision.

20

Using a Helpful Tone of Voice

Oh what it is that makes me tremble so as voices?
Surely whoever speaks to me in the right voice,
him or her I shall follow.
—WALT WHITMAN

Speaking with a pleasant tone of voice helps you to have harmonious relations with ill people. Your voice by itself can turn people on or off. Communications research indicates that a person's voice can be five times more important than the words he or she utters. This is something to be aware of when speaking with someone who is sick.

Your voice sends messages in many ways, including by its tone, pitch, variation, rate, and emphasis on certain words and phrases. And people make judgments about you based on your voice characteristics. For example, if you speak in a high-pitched voice, people may surmise that you are excited, nervous, or insecure. If you speak softly or hesitantly, people may infer that you are uncertain about what you are saying.

Undesirable voice characteristics are a disadvantage—a distinct minus when you are conversing with a sick person. By speaking with a calm, unhurried voice at a low pitch, you encourage the ill person with whom you are talking to feel calm and serene. Try to speak naturally, with a pleasant tone. But be sure to sound like yourself, rather than adopting an overly soothing and reassuring tone of voice. Your tone and volume can be a help in conveying your concern and compassion for an ill individual.

There are several things to avoid when you are speaking with an ill person, because they typically create antagonism and resentment:

- A tonal inflection that sounds superior or condescending
- A preachy, scolding, holier-than-thou voice
- A sarcastic tone
- A tone of finality—your word is the last word on the subject
- A self-important, demanding tone
- An authoritarian, commanding tone
- A hurried or hesitant rate of speech
- A monotone—it suggests you're bored

It is important to recognize that how you say something generally has an even greater impact than what you are actually saying to the person. It is also wise to get honest feedback from people about the affects of your voice. Such feedback can be very beneficial; many people have an abrasive or offensive tone of voice that serves only to create resentment—yet tragically, they never realize it.

21

Using Body Language

*Language which does not acknowledge the body
does not acknowledge life.*

—JOHN LAHR

Most of us are unaware of the important role our bodies play in the way we communicate. Yet experience indicates that people communicate more than 50 percent of meaning through their body language. Your actual words send only a small portion of your message; most of your message is transmitted by your voice and body language.

Try to become more conscious of how your body language affects other people. The way you use your body will cause a positive or negative reaction in others, depending upon the interpretation made by the person with whom you are talking, and upon the particular situation.

Whenever you are talking with an ill person, be sure your body language is sending the right signals, and sending them clearly. For example, you may be creating a negative reaction merely by your facial expressions, your tone of voice, your gestures—even by the way you sit.

By using your body in the following ways, you can create a favorable reaction from someone who is ill:

- Talk at a distance comfortable for the other person: neither too close nor too far. If you get too close, you may make the other person think you are intrusive or pushy. But if you stand or sit too far away, you may give the impression you are cold and impersonal. It is important to realize that each of us has a distance comfort zone (a space bubble). Although this distance varies from person to person, generally twenty-four to forty inches is a good talking distance for most people. A distance as close as eighteen inches can be an acceptable distance for close friends and family.
- Sit in a relaxed manner, rather than on the edge of your chair.
- Be close enough to speak easily, without needing to raise your voice.
- Be able to see all the person without having any objects between you (e.g., a large vase).
- Face the person at his or her eye level, so that he or she doesn't need to strain his or her neck to see you.
- Make your facial expressions match what you are saying or hearing.
- Act relaxed, though not excessively so.
- Use frequent gestures, and move your body often, in a manner responsive to what you are saying and hearing.

- Maintain steady eye contact, without appearing to stare. Try not to noticeably look at your watch or a clock.
- Nod your head at appropriate times, to show that you are paying attention and that you understand what the person is saying.
- Smile fully and frequently—avoid partial, fleeting smiles.
- Lean forward toward the person, with an interested look on your face, while you are listening.
- Keep your arms and legs in a comfortable position (e.g., don't act tense by keeping your arms rigidly crossed, or restless by frequently moving your legs and feet).
- Match the tone of your voice to the words you are saying.
- Touch the person periodically, in appropriate ways, in order to convey caring and warmth (e.g., hold hands, give hugs, give shoulder rubs).

It is important to realize that your body is always saying something. You can shut off your words at will, but you can't ever shut off your body language. Consequently, it is wise to become more aware of exactly what your body is communicating to others at all times.

PART 2

HELPING

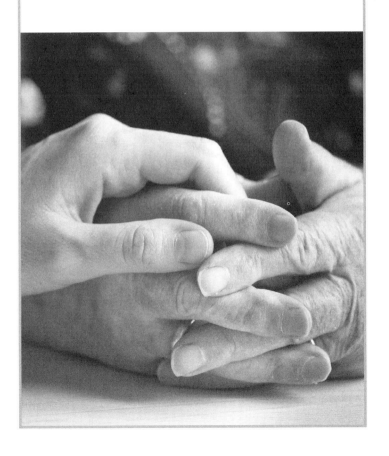

22

Being Available

Friendship, like love, is destroyed by long absence.
—SAMUEL JOHNSON

It is imperative that you be available to an ill person when he or she needs you. Simply *being there* is vital. There is no substitute for your physical presence.

In particular, do your best to be available when the sick person's needs are the greatest. Such times include times when he or she is

- In pain or considerable discomfort
- Frightened
- Upset
- Unable to sleep
- Depressed
- Is frightened after having just received bad news about his or her condition

Although your presence is crucial, don't feel guilty if you can't always be there physically for the person, or if you can't always be in the right frame of mind to be receptive to what the individual is saying. This is impossible, and it's not expected of you. Remember—you're only human, and you have your own limitations as well as your own needs.

Availability has two dimensions:
1. Accessibility
2. Approachability

Accessibility involves physical presence. It is important that you realize that your presence, not your words, means the most to the ill person. Your presence alone can be enough to show your concern for a friend or loved one; it is not always necessary for you to say or do something. Talk is not always needed—and sometimes simply sitting with the person is more desirable than talking because your talking can be a strain to a person who is in pain or who has only limited energy.

Make sure to emphasize to the ill person that you *want* to be present, and that you are eager to help. And make it very clear that your being there is in no way an imposition upon your time. Explain that you know that if your roles were reversed, the sick person would reciprocate, and would be there for you.

Be sure to also be approachable—be a mentally receptive, attentive listener who responds appropriately to whatever an ill individual tells you. Until you are both accessible and approachable, you are not truly available.

23

Being Caring

*What is done for those whom we care about becomes
a matter of one's personal pleasure, hard to express,
perhaps, but surely deeply felt.*
—Barrett Wendell

It is important to be a caring person. However, it is
equally important to realize that it is not enough to care
for an ill person—you must also demonstrate this caring
by your words and actions.

All of us need to feel cared for, and to feel that we are
valued as a person. All people want to feel appreciated,
respected, and held in high regard. This is especially true
for those who are chronically ill.

Empathy is a key ingredient in caring for someone.
Empathy involves doing your best to feel things as the ill
person feels them. Although you can't actually experience
things exactly the same way, you can identify what the
person is feeling. Recognize that empathy and sympathy
are different. Sympathy is simply feeling sorry for the other
person and his or her problems. Ill people need and want
your empathy—not your sympathy.

You care for someone when you are interested in him or her as a person. You face and share his or her problems with him or her. You are also concerned about his or her well-being. Furthermore, you feel a compassionate, non-possessive warmth toward the person.

A caring person wants to do the right things to help and to protect an ill person. He or she adapts to the ill person's needs. Caring for and wanting to help do not mean that you should take over and solve the person's problems for him or her. This is an unreasonable expectation; it is impossible for you to have the answers to all a sick person's problems.

As emphasized earlier, you need to show the sick person that you care about him or her. There are several things that you can say and do to demonstrate your caring. Some of the most important include

- Making ongoing comments to bolster the person's self-esteem and feelings of worth and value
- Giving of yourself by putting the sick person first and devoting a liberal amount of time to being present with the person and helping him or her
- Offering to help, and actually helping in meaningful ways
- Accepting what the person says and does, to the best of your ability
- Getting on the same wavelength by talking about the things the sick person wants to talk about, listening attentively, and then responding appropriately to what has been said

- Speaking in a warm, gentle tone of voice, at a rate easily understood by the other person
- Selecting your words carefully, using easy-to-understand language, and avoiding inflammatory words that upset the ill individual (but being careful not to talk down to the person)
- Speaking frequently of your love and affection for the person
- Exhibiting kind, loving facial expressions while interacting
- Sitting close to the person, and periodically touching them using appropriate patting, stroking, and rubbing
- Maintaining a relaxed, open body position
- Mirroring the person's body movements to show compatibility
- Being gracious when the person declines your offers to help with something (thus showing respect for the person's need for independence)
- Listening to the person discuss sensitive matters, such as spiritual things and feelings of futility or helplessness
- Refraining from saying or doing things that annoy or irritate the person (e.g., wearing offensive perfume or talking about controversial topics)

By saying and doing the things listed, as well as other similar things, you will be able to demonstrate your caring in specific, tangible ways. Remember how the word *care* stands for the key components of the act of caring:

C = compassion
A = acceptance
R = respect
E = empathy

24

Being Helpful

People seldom refuse help, if one offers it in the right way.
—A. C. BENSON

You are very important to a chronically ill person. Your help may be necessary for the well-being, even the life, of the person. Thus, it is advisable to think ahead of time about

- How you can help
- How much help the person really needs
- How much you are able to help, and how to explain your limits to the person who is ill

Much as you may want to give infinite help, there must be limits. The reality is that you have only so much you can give. You, too, have needs, regardless of how great the needs of the ill person may be.

It is important not to force your ideas for helping on the sick individual, who may view his or her needs differently. For example, you may want to help the person as much as possible, whereas he or she may wish to be helped as little as possible. It is unwise to be too insistent with offers to help based only on your own desires to help.

All your help should be motivated by the desire to help the person have a better life. What really matters is not what you want, or what you think is best, but what the sick person wants and thinks is best for him or her (if it isn't ill advised).

Typically the primary needs of an ill person include

- Being viewed as a person first, and an ill person second
- Having control of his or her life—having a feeling of being in charge
- Maintaining his or her feeling of self-esteem and value as a person
- Having the opportunity to state his or her views and have them respected
- Feeling accepted and appreciated for who he or she is
- Feeling safe and secure
- Having a sense of belonging and togetherness
- Being involved in important family events
- Having the freedom to do things on his or her own as much as possible
- Feeling loved and needed

Even a critically ill or dying person needs to feel that he or she still has the power to control his or her life. He or she wants to make the decisions about how he or she lives—as much as his or her condition permits. For example, he or she may wish to make decisions about

- What to eat, and when to eat it
- What to wear
- When to sleep, when to get up, and when to go to bed
- Where to spend his or her waking hours (e.g., bed, chair)
- How he or she wants his or her room arranged
- In what family doings or decisions he or she wants to be included

Any efforts, no matter how well intended, to spare a chronically ill person from family problems or difficult decisions may create feelings of isolation, resentment, and rejection. Regrettably, accepting help may be the only way the chronically ill person may have of conserving enough energy and strength to get through the day. Even in such situations, accepting help may be extremely difficult for a person who has enjoyed living an independent life, and being responsible for his or her own actions and decisions.

Thus, you must be willing to assist the person as indirectly as possible, and to avoid taking control of his or her life. It is best to develop the attitude *I'm willing to help you as little or as much as you want me to, but I won't do things for you that you prefer to do for yourself.* Follow the iron rule: "Never do for others what they can and should do for themselves."

There is no single prescribed way to help all people in all situations. Each person is different, and each situation is different; consequently, each person must be treated differently.

Thus, you need to be flexible and "play it by ear." Ask how you can help best, rather than presuming that you know. Sometimes a person may be in desperate need of help but, because of his or her pride, refuses to ask for help. In such a situation, you must sense the person's need for help and subtly offer help. You can also make suggestions of ways you can help. If your suggestion is declined, go ahead and make a couple of other suggestions in a low-key manner, but be aware when it is best to stop making any suggestions. It is a mistake to make too many suggestions, but also a mistake to always wait to be asked for help.

If you want to be of assistance but don't know how to be, simply ask the ill person how you can help. Be careful not to be too demanding; always give the person the option to refuse your offer.

A general offer to help is, in essence, an offer to do nothing. Take, for example, a quick, off-hand comment: "Let me know if I can help." It's like "Let's do lunch sometime"— nothing generally happens unless your offer is specific.

In situations in which the person is capable of making decisions completely by himself or herself, you can ask questions such as these:

- "What if this were to happen?"
- "How would you feel if you were to . . . ?"
- "What would you like to wear today?"
- "Would you prefer beans for your vegetable tonight, or peas?"
- "Where would you like the flowers?"

There are four kinds of mistakes you may make when giving help:

1. Giving advice without considering whether it is appropriate for the person and situation
2. Trying to help the person at the wrong time
3. Being too assertive, causing the ill person to become resistant and defensive
4. Trying to help a person who doesn't want to be helped

Try to resist the temptations to offer advice, or solve the person's problems, by saying unhelpful things such as

- "If I were you I would . . ."
- "This will be good for you."
- "Believe me—this is what you should do."
- "My best advice to you is . . ."
- "Trust me I know what is best for you."

These kinds of statements can make the person feel helpless and dependent—perhaps even manipulated.

Sometimes you may need to help an ill person solve a problem. Go ahead, but be sure you listen fully to the person's explanation of the problem before you begin to discuss how to solve it. Also, be careful not to take over the problem. When considering a solution, focus on the person's feelings as well as the facts related to the problem. And face reality—not all problems have solutions, so don't feel obligated to have the answers to everything. It's perfectly all right to say, "I don't know" or "I'm sorry, but I can't do that."

In your sincere desire to help the person, you may be inclined to make instant or ill-advised promises, a tendency that can cause problems. Your pledged word must be sacred and honored, so when it comes to making promises, be sure you

- Keep your promises
- Refrain from making promises you can't keep
- Apologize when you can't fulfill a promise, and honestly explain why you became unable to do so; see if you can substitute something else satisfactory for the thing promised

We all have problems and feel the need to discuss them at times, but when you are discussing an ill person's problems, resist the temptation to interject your own and discuss them at length. It is fine to share your problems briefly, to build a spirit of togetherness, but do so infrequently, and whenever you do so, share only in bite-sized chunks. Never share to excess.

It is a good idea to periodically reassure the ill person of your genuine desire to help, assuring him or her that he or she is important to you, that you enjoy helping him or her and that in no way is doing so an imposition on you.

It is crucial that you understand that "help" is not always helpful. Sometimes, an attempt to help can be harmful. Your challenge is to be ever mindful of when helping is helpful and when it is harmful.

25

Being Natural

What is natural is never disgraceful.
—Euripides

Most people are uncomfortable around chronically ill people; many times they don't know what to say or do. But it is best to simply be the real you—in your appearance, in your words, and in your actions. You enhance your relations with ill people when you are natural, genuine, and authentic. But you make a person suspicious and endanger your relations with him or her when you play a role, hide behind a façade, or mask your real feelings. People respect you when you act as you really are, but they are uncomfortable around phonies and don't respect them.

Those who are chronically ill can readily detect pretentious, phony behavior. And when they do, they wonder what your purpose is, and why you don't act like your true self.

By being genuine and real, you help someone who is ill express his or her true thoughts and feelings. He or she feels that because you are acting sincere and real, he or

she can reciprocate by being natural and sincere
with you.

When your behavior appears natural, spontaneous,
and free of deception, it makes someone who is ill feel
more relaxed, and less defensive, around you. He or she
doesn't feel a need to be on guard constantly. When you
are open and straightforward with someone who is sick, he
or she, in turn, can be open and honest with you.

Just be yourself. Act and talk like you really care. If you
are generally an optimistic, upbeat person, act that way
around someone who is sick—being sensitive to his or her
mood, of course. But trying to put on a show of cheerfulness when you don't really feel that way will be readily
detected by an ill person as nothing more than contrived.
Ill people have sensitive antennae and are generally more
adept at reading peoples' behavior than you might realize.

When you are talking with someone who is chronically ill, make yourself feel genuinely relaxed and at ease.
Be comfortable to be with. You will feel less nervous if you
realize that your presence and support are the things that
really count, not your ability to answer every question or
solve all problems.

During your conversations with someone who is ill,
center on the person rather than being preoccupied with
recommended techniques for dealing with ailing people.
Having the proper attitude about someone who is sick is
much more important than using a particular technique
for dealing with them. It can't be overemphasized: an ill

person is first of all a person—a real person to care about, not a case to treat.

Use words that sound like you, and not somebody else. Don't try to sound like a preacher, doctor, or therapist. Say what you believe needs to be said, and do it in a kindly manner. Avoid playing games by overpoliteness, excessive concern, or extreme solicitousness.

Allow yourself to spontaneously gesture and move your body normally. Touch when it is natural to do so, rather than planning for or contrived times to do so. Be flexible; adapt what you say and do to the needs of the moment. Let common sense be your guide.

Let your hair down, and don't hesitate to show your real feelings. Act the way you really want to act. Speak from deep within yourself, and share your real thoughts; for example, express your real concerns without fearing to show tenderness.

At night, when you look in the mirror after visiting with someone who is chronically ill, like what you see, and respect yourself for having acted natural and honest when you were with a person who was sick.

26

Being Nonconfrontational

If thou faint in the day of adversity, thy strength is small.
—PROVERBS 24:10

Normally it is best to avoid confrontation with a chronically sick person. It is wise to limit confrontation to important matters—for example, some matter endangering the ill person's health, or something that could jeopardize the family's well-being. The sad fact is that confrontation is sometimes necessary, even inescapable. But it makes sense to try to avoid confronting an ill person over minor problems or issues—instead, overlook them, and move on.

You confront someone when you demand an explanation for something that a person said or did. You also confront someone whenever you insist that a person give you reasons to justify something done, or not done, to which you object.

Confrontation includes such things as
- Having a face-to-face encounter over a clash of opinions

- Calling a person to task, in an emotional manner, over something you disagree with
- Challenging a person boldly over something
- Expressing opposing views defiantly

Confrontation frequently becomes heated when you confront in an aggressive manner. This causes the other party to feel cornered and threatened—and to reciprocate in kind.

It must be emphasized that you want to limit confrontation to only the most serious matters—for example, refusing to take essential medicine, or actions creating family friction.

You can usually avoid confrontation by doing the following:

- Analyze your own communication style. If it is too aggressive, tone it down.
- Be polite in all you say, and courteous in all you do.
- Be more accepting, and less judgmental.
- Carefully digest what you hear, and refrain from making immediate, off-the-top-of-your-head responses.
- Say things calmly, and in a low-pitched voice.
- Use neutral language and noninflammatory words.
- Refuse to get upset by the other person's use of words that you find objectionable.
- Avoid discussing certain topics about which either of you has strong feelings.

- Refrain from the use of sarcasm, ridicule, and undue criticism.
- Control your emotions when listening to something with which you strongly disagree.
- Try to view things from the other person's viewpoint.
- Meet issues indirectly, rather than head-on (e.g., "We seem to differ on how to solve your eating problem—how do you think we can resolve our differences?").
- Permit the other person to control things, rather than your trying to dominate and run things.
- Allow the person to have his or her own opinions and beliefs without trying to force him or her to adopt yours. Remember: "A person persuaded against his will is of the same opinion still."
- Predict possible objections and reactions to what you contemplate saying or doing.

However, as mentioned earlier, it is sometimes necessary to confront an ill person. If confrontation is required and you refuse to act, you are being irresponsible, unwise, and perhaps even cowardly.

The following approaches have proven successful when confronting someone:

- Confront positively, and with a desire to be helpful.
- Be compassionate in all that you say and do.
- Confront in a low-key manner—avoid being pushy.
- Mirror the person's statements when he or she

is upset; for example, "You feel as though I have mistreated you."

- Listen much more than you talk.
- Offer the main reasons for your viewpoint, without engaging in overkill.
- Phrase what you have to say tactfully, so that what you say is less offensive to the other person.
- Make your point clearly—but once you've made it, move on.
- Help the person to save face; provide him or her with an honorable out. For example, you might say, "I realize you were in pain and probably didn't mean everything you said."
- Avoid presenting your views and reasons too vigorously, as this invites an equally vigorous response.
- Try to agree in principle, to agree on what you disagree on, or to agree to disagree whenever you can't agree on something even after a prolonged discussion.

The "I perceive" technique can minimize the risk of confrontation. When you use this proven technique, say things such as

- "As I see it . . ."
- "In my viewpoint . . ."
- "Now this is only my opinion—I could be wrong."

In essence, when you use the "I perceive" approach, you are merely explaining how things look to you. This is usually much more acceptable to the other person than your stating categorically *this is the way things are—period.*

The main benefits of the "I perceive" approach are that it

- Minimizes emotion
- Is less threatening to the other party
- Allows you to honestly state your perceptions of something, but in a less stinging manner
- States what you believe without placing any fault or blame; thus, there is no need for the person being confronted to become defensive

It is important to note that it is improper to use the "I perceive" technique when definite facts are available. You should say, for example, "The chart recording your medicines shows that you have not been taking your medicines regularly—this is a serious matter, and I need you to tell me why."

In addition, there are symptoms of resistance to your efforts to confront of which you should be aware:

- Nervous laughter
- Long pauses, or tense responses to what you've said
- Attempts to change the subject
- Fast, furious talk in opposition
- Reticence, sullenness, or insolence
- Withdrawal—for example, "I need to sleep now" or "I'm too tired to discuss anything right now"

The causes of resistance to your attempts to confront typically include any of a variety of reasons:

- The other person dislikes the topic so much, or is so embarrassed, that he or she refuses to talk about it.
- Your approach is ineffective:
- You sound intimidating, or as if you are an interrogator.
- You overwhelm the person with too much talk.
- You appear to be giving unwanted advice, or to be excessively urging.
- The other person mistrusts your motives.
- The other person expects to be criticized or censured.

Sometimes during a confrontation, despite your best efforts, the person becomes angry. In such an instance, follow these steps:

- Listen carefully, and control your own emotions.
- Refrain from interrupting.
- Remain silent until the person calms down and is ready to listen to you.
- Mirror the person's statements, without any attempt to interpret or rephrase them.
- Explain your position, calmly and at a measured pace.
- Discontinue your explanation if the person becomes angry again and refuses to listen to you. If this happens, you could say something like, "I don't think now is a good time to pursue this further. Let's wait until we can both think about this some more and then talk again, okay?"

- Try to discuss the matter later, when the heat has subsided and you think the person is ready to listen.
- If the delay isn't successful, you could say something like, "I can see you don't want to discuss your need to take your medicine with me, so let's wait until your doctor has a chance to talk to you about the problem."

Remember: confrontation may be unpleasant, but it may occasionally be necessary. However, you will be wise to limit such occasions as much as you can. There is no point in upsetting or alienating the other person unless conditions make it absolutely unavoidable.

27

Counseling

He that will not be counseled cannot be helped.
—John Clarke

The chronically ill person typically has problems that trouble him or her, and that need to be discussed. He or she may feel lonely, isolated, and depressed. He or she may feel anxious about the future, worrying that he or she is losing control of his or her life. Someone who is chronically ill frequently needs help to deal with these problems.

Counseling is a method to help people understand and overcome their problems—or at least learn to live with them.

There are three basic approaches to counseling of which you need to be aware:

1. The directive approach: Essentially, tell the person how to solve his or her problems.
2. The semidirective approach: Help the person identify the different options for solving his or her problems, and offer some advice.

3. The nondirective approach: Rely on the person to solve his or her own problems as a result of discussing them with you.

The best approach to use usually depends on three things:
1. Your counseling knowledge and ability
2. The personality and ability of the person being counseled
3. The nature and severity of the problem

Irrespective of the counseling approach you decide to use, it is imperative that you proceed with caution. An important part of being an effective counselor is knowing your limitations, and knowing what to do, and not do, as well as when, and when not, to do it.

Do your best to observe these cautions when counseling any ill person:
- Insist that the person own the problem and take responsibility himself or herself for solving it.
- Recognize that you can't (and shouldn't) solve someone else's problems, or try to have all the answers for another's problems.
- Show compassion for the person with the problem, but remain objective about the problem itself.
- Realize that the person must be willing to be helped and must have a sincere desire to be counseled by you concerning the problem, or your efforts will fail.

- Refrain from acting judgmentally or jumping to conclusions before the problem is adequately identified.
- Make clear what you are, and are not, willing to do in your role as counselor.

Your primary responsibilities as a counselor are
- To be supportive and show that you care
- To listen to the person express his or her thoughts and feelings
- To help him or her clarify his or her thoughts and feelings about the problem
- To help him or her feel better about the problem

Although most ill people have the potential to profit from counseling, you can't realistically expect easy solutions to problems or sudden drastic changes in troubled behavior.

In your role as counselor, you can choose different levels of lead when helping people solve their problems, but it is generally best, and safest, to use the least degree of lead possible. The levels of lead from least to most are

1. Simply listen in an interested, permissive, nondirective manner, without saying anything.
2. Make accepting, supportive comments occasionally, such as these: "I see," "Uh huh," and "I understand."
3. Restate what the person has said, without saying anything new, merely mirroring what the person has said.

4. Clarify what the person said using slightly different words from those actually said, or by asking questions to clear up anything you didn't understand.
5. Summarize periodically what the person has said, to promote overall understanding.
6. Introduce new ideas in a neutral fashion; for example, "what do you think of this idea?"
7. Interpret what the person has said; for example, "What you have said about wanting to slow down your exercises will mean that it will take you longer to build up your strength."
8. Give advice or urge a specific course of action; for example, "If I were you, this is what I would do."

If your counseling endeavors are to succeed, the ill person must trust you and feel safe with you. He or she must feel confident that you will hold everything he or she tells you in strictest confidence. Also, you must foster a warm, permissive climate that puts the ill person at ease, and that encourages him or her to express his or her thoughts and feelings freely and fully.

Conversely, your counseling cannot succeed unless you avoid

- Having a preconceived notion of what the real problem is
- Making judgments based on your own values, or moralizing

- Stating your own views of the problem, or becoming too actively involved
- Taking over the problem and solving it for the person
- Telling the person what to do, or offering strong advice
- Acting like a parent dealing with a child, rather than discussing the problem as equal adults
- Talking more than you listen
- Downplaying or minimizing the problem with remarks such as, "You're making a mountain out of a molehill" or "Things are not as bad as they seem"
- Discussing the problem before discovering what it really is
- Minimizing the person's feelings about the problem and stressing only the facts of the problem
- Holding the discussion at the wrong time or in the wrong place
- Acting impatient or irritable over the sick person's thought process

Here are a couple of additional thoughts to consider when helping an ill person with his problems:
- A person often knows the right thing to do, but does not want to do it.
- People do what they do the way they do it because of who they are.

28

Leveling With Someone

Whenever anyone has anything unpleasant to say,
one should always be quite candid.
—OSCAR WILDE

Leveling is necessary when speaking to someone who is chronically ill. You are doing a disservice to someone who is sick when you fail to provide him or her with important information. You must say what must be said, even though what you have to say may not always be welcome. Leveling with someone, particularly if he or she is ill, is not easy. In fact, it can be extremely hard. Leveling requires courage, and it requires the ability to be candid with people. It also involves the possible risk of alienating the other person if what you have to tell him or her is unpleasant or critical in nature.

When you level with someone, you say what is on your mind, honestly, candidly, directly, and in a straightforward manner. You say clearly what needs to be said, leaving no doubt in the other person's mind about what you've said. When you level, get directly to the point, without being abrupt. Focus on the ill person's needs rather than your own, but never apologize for the need to level, and don't be overly polite, lest you do your message a disservice by weakening it.

Before leveling, assure the person that you intend only to be helpful. Explain to him or her how he or she will benefit from your comments. Because leveling involves sharing important information about a serious matter, it is essential that you realize that leveling can be about something positive as well as negative—in other words, it can involve both praise and criticism.

Try to level about the issue without leveling the person in the process; in no way does "leveling" imply that you can say anything you want, irrespective of the consequences, or that you can let the person have it with both barrels. It is unwise to simply dump on the person, or to overload the person with too much information at one time—instead, address only one major issue at a time. Once you've made your point and it has been understood, move on rather than dwelling on the matter. While leveling, be objective about the facts and compassionate about the person; try to act more like a coach than a judge throughout the discussion.

Before leveling with anyone, do your homework. Be sure that you have all the facts, and that you have them straight. Additionally, it is best to level about behavior and conditions that can be changed. It is not fair to hold a person accountable for things he or she cannot control.

Focus on a person's specific behavior, and not the total person; for example, you might note that the person's overall cooperation is wonderful, and worthy of commendation, but that his or her cooperation on personal hygiene leaves much to be desired, and must be discussed frankly. It is crucial that you be as reasonable and objective as possible throughout the entire leveling process.

Tell the truth, the whole truth, and nothing but the truth. The ill person is entitled to all the truth, honestly presented. Refrain from being overly protective by omitting, understating, or exaggerating the facts. Say what needs to be said, simply and plainly. Don't hedge your comments, and avoid qualifying your statements with "weasel words" such as *perhaps* and *maybe*. Be judicious with the use of euphemisms, lest they weaken the point you are trying to make.

When you level, be confident, and take control of the situation, without any hint of arrogance. Be relaxed, and try to put the person you are leveling with at ease as much as the situation permits. Reduce as much tension as possible, so that the person will be less defensive and more receptive to what you have to say. Speak in a conversational tone and with a pleasant manner (yet with a serious demeanor). Accept responsibility for your comments by using *I* statements rather than *they* statements. Speak for yourself.

You can improve your chances of securing a favorable reaction if you match your approach to the ill person's personality. Tailoring your comments to the individual is a must. For example, with some people, it is better to proceed directly to the point; with others, it is better to lead into the point indirectly. And it is always a good idea to explain exactly how the person can profit from what you are going to tell him or her. Be certain to talk *with* the person, and not *at* him or her; make suggestions, rather than demands, about the issue at hand.

Leveling is best viewed as a sharing process. To be effective, it needs to be a two-way interaction. Your leveling attempt will be more successful if your past behavior has shown that you yourself are willing to be leveled with. Such reciprocity adds credibility to the leveling proceedings.

Let's review several specific things you can do when leveling with someone that should enhance your prospects for success:

- Limit negative leveling to important and serious matters that require it.
- Allow sufficient time—it can't be rushed.
- Look assured, and be confident without being overbearing.
- Look directly at the person with a steady gaze, ready to observe instant feedback.
- Select a quiet, private place.
- Emphasize that everything said is in confidence.
- Face the issue—don't stall or ramble.
- Present the facts candidly, but as gently and tactfully as you can.

- Be as clear, explicit, and specific as possible.
- Select your words carefully. Avoid using words such as *failure*, *mistake*, and *wrong*. Also refrain from making statements such as "You should have known better," "I have warned you repeatedly about this," and "I can't believe you did such a stupid thing."
- Explain your position, and the reasoning behind it. Then listen to the person's response, keeping an open mind. Next, exchange views candidly (but don't argue).
- Try to gain agreement on the fact that a problem does exist, as well as an understanding of precisely what the problem is.
- Verify at the end of the discussion that the person not only understands the problem but that he or she also understands what, specifically, must be done about it.
- Close the discussion on a friendly note.
- Whenever you level, say what you mean, mean what you say, and don't be mean when you say it.

Remember to keep a level playing field when leveling. It is as important to level about good behavior and good news as it is about bad behavior and bad news.

29

Timing

Ah! The clock is always slow: it is later than you think.
—Robert W. Service

Be aware of the times an ill person needs to talk with you, needs to be with you without any conversation, or wants to be alone. When together, learn to be comfortable with periods of silence. Many times, your simple presence is all a sick individual needs. In such instances, let the person be silent rather than pressuring him or her to talk, or feeling compelled to say something yourself.

It is wise to keep your visits brief, rather than prolonged. Frequent visits make it easier to maintain rapport, and to recall recent conversations. Short visits are also less tiring for the sick person.

Limit how much you say at any one time. You don't want to overload or overwhelm the person with too much information given all at once. It is hard for anyone to absorb and understand great amounts of information at one time—especially someone who is ailing. It is best to spread difficult-to-comprehend information over a period of time to help the person digest it; just like food, information is best digested in small bites. Sometimes you may need to repeat hard-to-understand information several times, stating the information in different ways, to attain understanding.

Occasionally, ill people talk for extended periods of time at night about things concerning them that they never mention in daytime. This is because people tend to be less inhibited, revealing more of what is on their mind, when they are tired and when their defenses are down. They are also more likely to speak frankly when they are feeling irritated and upset.

Try to talk about important things at the best time for the chronically ill person, rather than the most convenient time for you. It is helpful to know the activities the person was involved in immediately before your visit, and those in which he or she will be engaged immediately after your visit; competing activities can significantly affect a person's receptivity to what you have to say.

It is important to talk about anything important when the ill person's mind is clear, and when he or she is in the right mood to listen to what you have to say. It is also a good idea to know when and when not to convey important information; you can do this by sizing up a person's mood. If he or she doesn't appear to be paying attention, or his or her reactions aren't conducive to get-ting your message across and acted upon, it may be wise to stop talking, and to postpone any further comments for a more opportune time. There is no question that timing is crucial to the successful exchange of important information.

Do your best to share important information promptly, but be sure to take the necessary time to get all the facts, and to get them straight, before sharing the information. Talk slowly enough to be clear, and to make certain you are understood (you can ensure you have been understood by getting feedback). If the information is sensitive or confidential, talk at a time and place that guarantees privacy. If the news you are going to share is extremely happy or sad, consider having other appropriate people present to share the moment.

By selecting the best time, and most favorable conditions, for sharing vital information, you increase the chances that your message will be well received. Consider these tips to enhance the response to important information you need to share:

- Share information at the best time of day for the ailing person. Know whether he or she is a morning or night person.
- Do it when the person is rested, not sleepy or drowsy.
- Do it when the person is not hungry, nor groggy from a recently eaten meal.
- Do it when no significant event has immediately preceded, or will immediately follow, the time you plan to convey the information.

- Do it when the person is most alert, neither preoccupied or withdrawn.
- Do it when the person is as free of pain as possible.
- Do it when the negative affect of the person's medicine is minimal.
- Do it when your relationship is harmonious, free of strain or tension.
- Do it when the area is quiet and free of distraction.
- Do it when the person is in a good mood.
- Do it when sufficient time is available, freeing you from having to rush.
- Do it when you are in a positive frame of mind.

When you have vital information to share with an ill individual, it is imperative that you pick the best time to do it. Your timing could make the difference between a successful exchange of information and an unsuccessful one.

30

Touching Helpfully

He wants the natural touch.
—William Shakespeare

Know the power of touching. Touch is the most powerful of all the methods of communicating. A touch can say more than a million words. It is clear that all of us, well and sick alike, need the comfort and reassurance of physical contact.

Being seriously ill is a frightening experience for most people. It often causes strong feelings of insecurity, loneliness, and isolation. These feelings occur because many people stay away from sick people, not knowing what to say or do around them. Sick people are often an unsolved mystery to friends and loved ones alike.

When you touch an ailing person, you are saying, "You are not alone; I am here with you." Holding a person's hand, kissing his or her cheek, giving a hug, or patting an arm can be extremely comforting to a person who feels afraid and lonely. Conversely, your words have less impact on a person who is seriously ill.

Most people like it, and those who are chronically ill in particular, when friends and loved ones come close to them physically. Being close and touching are the best ways of showing a person that he or she is loved, cared for, and safe.

The appropriate way to touch an ill person depends on the closeness of your relationship with him or her, and his or her willingness to be touched. When you touch the person, be certain that he or she wants to be touched by you. Be sensitive to the person's response to your touching. If he or she gives even the slightest indication that he or she doesn't want to be touched, stop immediately. Make sure you don't invade his or her space bubble (the person's distance comfort zone). On the other hand, if you stay too far away from the sick person, you may be communicating that you don't want to be close to him or her, thus increase his or her feelings of separation and isolation.

Always be careful that you touch the person in the proper manner, and only in appropriate places. Make sure that your touching is not misinterpreted. It is normally acceptable to touch a person by

- Holding the person's hand
- Putting a hand on, or squeezing, an arm or shoulder
- Touching an elbow
- Patting a shoulder or the upper back
- Rubbing the back
- Giving tender hugs
- Giving a quick kiss on the cheek

Your touching should be a natural, spontaneous gesture of caring, rather than something planned or contrived.

Touching in appropriate ways clearly demonstrates your compassion and caring for the person. It helps you to connect better and promotes a feeling of togetherness. There is something about the act of touching that helps a seriously ill person feel safe, and more willing to open up and talk more freely with you. Your touching tends to create greater trust, and to break down the person's inhibitions.

The affect of your touching on the ill person depends on the following factors:

- The type of your relationship (e.g., parent, distant cousin)
- The closeness of your relationship (e.g., whether you see each other often, with mutually warm feelings, or infrequently, with only polite interaction)
- The part of the body you touch (e.g., face, hand)
- How long the touching lasts (e.g., fleeting, prolonged)
- How much pressure you exert (e.g., gentle touching of a shoulder, rubbing of a shoulder)

It is natural to touch a seriously ill person when greeting him or her, or when saying goodbye. A quick kiss on the cheek, the touching of an arm or shoulder, or a lingering handshake can do wonders when you are saying hello to a person. It is also comforting to touch the person periodically throughout the conversation. Touching is particularly important whenever the ill person is telling you about his or her aches and pains, describing his or her fears or problems, or explaining his or her feelings of loneliness or his or her regrets about being a burden on the family.

It cannot be overemphasized that the proper touching at appropriate times can mean the world to a chronically ill individual. There is simply no substitute for it.

PART 3

LISTENING AND OBSERVING

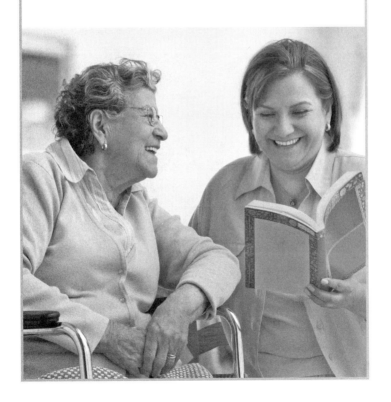

31

Hearing Someone Out

*A good listener tries to understand thoroughly
what the other person is saying. In the end he may
disagree sharply, but before he disagrees he wants
to know exactly what it is he is disagreeing with.*
—Kenneth Wells

Ill people need someone to listen to them. And they need unselfish listening, listening that focuses completely on what they are saying. Thus, it is vital that you show consideration for a sick person's need to talk, and to be listened to. Let the chronically ill person set the agenda, because he or she—and he or she alone—knows what he or she wishes to talk about. Topics discussed don't need to be in any particular order—just let the person express his or her thoughts and feelings spontaneously, as they come up.

An ill person needs to talk about topics of interest to him or her, such as daily events, family doings, and his or her condition, complaints, problems, hopes, and fears. He or she needs to be able to share with you his or her thoughts and feelings at the time.

Limit how much you yourself talk; the ill person's opportunity to talk is more important than yours. And remember this key point: if you are talking, you are not listening. To spend time with an ailing person most profitably, you need to be willing to use your time listening, and responding to what you hear.

When a sick person doesn't have ample opportunity to talk about his or her world, friends, and loved ones, he or she feels lonely and isolated, and may even feel resentful.

To hear a person out, you first need to clear your own mind of your problems and concerns. You can't listen well to an ill person if you are preoccupied with your own inner conflicts, or when your thinking is dominated by your own problems. Many ill people are perceptive enough to easily detect when you are preoccupied, and listening to them only to be polite. They need you to be with them completely, mentally as well as physically. Like anyone, someone who is ill resents it when you fake listening to him or her.

Try to listen with an open mind. Do your best to listen objectively, with a neutral rather than judgmental attitude. It is essential that you avoid prejudging or jumping to conclusions about what you hear—to do so is not only insensitive, but unfair, and it can sometimes be dangerous. It's wise to delay making any judgments until you've heard all the facts and feelings that are being expressed.

By concentrating completely on what an ailing individual is saying, and having a total commitment to hearing the person out, you can avoid a number of bad listening habits:

- Preparing what you are going to say next in your own mind when you should be listening to the person who is speaking
- Tuning out what the person is saying, because you believe you already know what he or she is going to say
- Arguing mentally with what the person is saying to you
- Listening in order to refute, rather than understand, what you hear
- Becoming distracted by certain words or phrases that cause you to become upset or agitated
- Becoming self-protective and defensive when you disagree with what you hear
- Hearing what you want, or expect, to hear, rather than what is actually being said
- Making premature judgments, and jumping to conclusions

Additionally, here are several tips you will find helpful when trying to hear a person out:

- Get relaxed, and make yourself comfortable.
- Listen patiently, without any hint of being in a rush.
- Encourage the person to say everything on his or her mind: "Won't you please tell me more?" "Is there anything else you want to tell me?"

- Let the person vent his or her feelings fully.
- Refrain from interrupting unless doing so is absolutely necessary.
- Minimize all distractions: before talking at length, ask permission to turn off the television or radio.
- Listen with complete attention. Don't daydream, don't take mental vacations, don't let your mind wander, and don't listen only in spurts.
- Listen attentively to the person until he or she has discussed the topic completely, to his or her satisfaction—don't change the subject prematurely or abruptly.
- Wait things out, even when the person is having difficulty expressing himself or herself. Don't substitute or supply words, and don't finish sentences when he or she pauses or hesitates.
- Use silence to your advantage; for instance, let emotionally charged or highly significant statements sink in before you respond.
- Keep the previous list of bad habits in your mind to avoid.

By having the right attitude, and saying and doing the right things, you will be able to hear a person out, and you will avoid hearing, "You never hear anything I say to you."

32

Observing Body Language

Trust not a man's words if you please,
or you may come to very erroneous conclusions;
but at all times place implicit confidence in a man's
countenance in which there is no deceit.
—GEORGE BORROW

You can seldom get the entire meaning of what anyone is saying only from the words he or she utters. You must also observe his or her body language. And when reading body language, it is essential that you realize that no single body sign has meaning by itself.

Like other people, those who are chronically ill have other ways of communicating than merely through words. They also talk to you through voice intonation and variation, pauses, facial expressions, gestures, and body posture and movement. Their body language can provide you with rich clues as to what they are really thinking and feeling.

Observing body language involves knowing what to look for as well as where to look for it and how to observe it. Accurate and dependable observation is possible only after you know a person well, and knowing a person well requires frequent contact, as well as the opportunity to observe his or her attitudes and behaviors in a variety of circumstances.

We all send mixed messages from time to time. Unintentionally, our words and body language sometimes contradict each other, which confuses the people with whom we are talking. Normally, we aren't aware that we are sending mixed messages while we are doing it.

When you receive a mixed message, you're better off paying more attention to the speaker's body language than to his or her words. This is because body language is hard to disguise and fake. And when you're uncertain about the real meaning of the mixed message, ask questions. You can feel most certain about the true meaning of a mixed message when a person's words, voice, and body movement all are sending the same message.

To observe body language, watch for the following indicators in various parts of the body:

Head and Face Indicators

A person's head movements and facial expressions probably convey his or her person's feelings most clearly. Different parts of the face give clues to different emotions. For example, fear is shown most clearly in the eyes, whereas anger is disclosed by the face, the brow, and the forehead.

Eye Indicators

Eyes are good indicators of people's feelings, both because people are less aware of what their eyes are doing and because it is hard to control or disguise eye movement.

Eye indicators include
blink rate
shifting gaze

Body Posture/Positioning Indicators

A person's body positions can convey a number of messages, including those communicating energy/fatigue, interest/boredom, like/dislike, approval/disapproval, anxiety/relaxation, and general attitude toward you.

Body positioning indicators include
sudden changes in position
turning toward or away from you
movement from side to side

Gestures

Both the frequency and the type of a person's gestures demonstrate his or her attitude in general as well as his or her feelings toward you. For example, frequent and free gestures generally signify a liking toward you as well as comfort with the situation. Relaxed, open palm gestures also indicate ease with you. Conversely, scarce and restricted gestures usually convey dislike of you or discomfort with a situation or a topic of conversation.

You read gestures by noticing the number, speed, timing, size (large or small) of the various gestures.

Hand and Arm Movement:

A person's hand and arm movements are very revealing, because they are typically spontaneous and are thus rarely inhibited. Observe

- Whether the arms are folded, or resting comfortably on the sides or in the lap
- When and how the hands and arms move
- Whether the hands are relaxed, or tapping or drumming restlessly

Leg and Foot Movement:

Leg and foot movement are also highly revealing because a person moves them naturally without thinking about it. Frequent shifting of leg positions and foot tapping commonly express feelings of restlessness and anxiety.

Notice if a person's legs are crossed, whether they are crossed toward or away from you. Crossed toward you is a positive indicator and crossed away from you is a negative indicator. Note if they are crossed in a relaxed manner. Also observe the frequency and timing of leg motion.

Proximity Indicators

A person communicates nonverbally through his or her proximity to you. Notice whether the person sits or stands close to or away from you. Also be aware of whether the person leans toward or away from you while talking with you.

Voice Indicators

A person's voice provides another nonverbal communication that discloses a good deal about his or her mood:

- Rate of speech—fast, moderate, slow or hesitant
- Pitch level—confident low key or high nervous sound
- Loudness—softer, louder, trailing off

There are several other points worth noting. These include the times ill people are reluctant, maybe even afraid, to say something about sensitive matters that are highly important to them. By studying their body language, you may be able to detect this even though the person's words provide no indication of this.

Most of all, it is important to recognize that sometimes strong feelings are conveyed better without words. We are communicating with our bodies whenever we are awake. Independent of our conscious choice, our bodies send messages all the time, and we can do nothing to prevent them. For example, even people who are near death and entirely unable to speak can still communicate in various ways—for example, by responding to questions through a series of eye blinks or by squeezing the hand.

- Note: Much of this book's information about body language is drawn from the writings of various authorities on the subject, including Robert Birdwhistell, Edward Hall, and Julius Fast.

33

Interpreting Body Language

*We have so many words for states of the mind
and so few for states of the body.*
—Jeanne Moreau

Interpreting body language is especially helpful when an ill person's verbal message is obscure, incomplete or garbled. But you need to be cautious when trying to read body language. It is imperative that you realize that no one single body sign has meaning by itself. It is both ill-advised and dangerous to make judgments based on your interpretation of only one body behavior. The reading of a pattern or a combination of body signals is a must—it is the only accurate, safe way of interpreting body language.

Any accurate interpretation of body language must include understanding of three things:

1. The context, or particular situation.
2. The person's ethnic background and culture.
3. The surrounding pattern of facial expressions and body movements.

Experts on kinesics (the study of body language) have identified certain facial expressions and body movements that generally indicate a person's attitudes and feelings. Again, although these interpretations are usually true, recognize that they do not apply to all individuals, all the time, in all situations. Here are several behaviors of which you need to be aware when reading body language:

Symptoms of Nervousness
picking/rubbing the flesh
scratching
chewing the lower lip
covering mouth with hand when speaking
fidgeting in bed or in a chair
looking down or away
rapidly blinking the eyes

Symptoms of Defensiveness
crossing the arms tightly across the chest
crossing the legs away from other person

Symptoms of Judgmentalism
tilting the head to one side
peering over the glasses
forming a pyramid with the hands
karate chops with the arms
stroking the chin
raising the eyebrows

Symptoms of Skepticism or Suspicion
crossing the arms
rubbing the nose
leaning back, away from other person

Symptoms of Frustration
taking short, quick breaths
wringing the hands
rubbing the back of the neck
sighing
rubbing hands in hair

Symptoms of Insecurity
pinching the flesh
looking down
chewing the lips
biting nails

Symptoms of Confidence
forming a steeple with the hands
steady eye contact
free, unrestricted arm and hand movements

Symptoms of Cooperativeness
upper body leaning forward
uncrossed arms and legs
head nodding up and down
relaxed body position

These are only a few examples of how you can interpret various body movements. (You will note that there is some overlap of the meaning of certain facial expressions or body movements.) As you get to know an ill person better and you both become more open and comfortable with each other, you will be in a better position to interpret the person's body language, and thus to communicate better.

34

Listening Between the Lines

*One friend, one person who is truly understanding,
who takes the trouble to listen to us as we consider our
problem, can change our whole outlook on the world.*
—Dr. Elton Mayo

We frequently hear a person's words without paying attention to their deeper meaning. Thus, we may hear what a person actually says but miss the real intent of what they were saying. Because of this, we must be alert to an ill person's implicit message as well as his or her explicit message.

Be willing to wrestle with the thorny problem of interpreting what a person is really trying to say to you. Listen to the feelings, as well as the facts, opinions, and ideas, expressed. Listen carefully both to what is said and to what is not said.

People do not always say exactly what they mean or mean exactly what they say. They often have difficulty talking candidly, freely, and clearly about their innermost feelings. The seriously ill especially need to be listened to carefully, because they want you to hear what they are not saying but would like to say. In reality, many ill people wear masks to conceal their real feelings, concerns, and fears. They would actually like to share their real feelings honestly with their friends and loved ones, but sometimes don't dare to do so. They dread exposing their fears and weaknesses and then having them misunderstood or rejected. Consequently, they frequently present a façade of confidence and assurance outside while trembling with uncertainty within.

You need to be intuitive to see behind these façades and to see and hear the real person. Listening between the lines requires great effort, as well as the use of all your senses. Your ears must be tuned in, your eyes must be watchful, your mind must be alert, your heart must be open, and your intuition must be turned on. All your senses must be on high alert.

Be sure to listen diligently to everything an ill person says to you—don't quickly dismiss any statement as irrelevant. Idle chatter and chit-chat may seem to be of little importance on the surface, but upon careful analysis they may be telling you something significant. Be sensitive to the fact that an ill person may at first be discussing a "safe topic" with you to test your mood, in order to determine your receptivity to discussing something of great importance to him or her.

Behind a topic being discussed there may be subtle clues indicating distress, depression—even desperation—that have nothing to do with what is actually being discussed. It is a good idea to ask questions to encourage the person to say what is bothering him or her if you sense something more is going on than what is being said. For example, you might say, "I sense there may be more behind what you're saying than what you're telling me right now. Why don't you tell me about it?" Listen carefully and perceptively to the answer. Many times seemingly irrational comments make sense when you understand what is behind them.

Do your best to be aware when something is different about how the sick person is talking or acting. To gain this awareness, you must center your full attention on the sick individual and give up any preoccupation with your own thoughts.

These tips will help you listen between the lines more effectively. Pay close attention to

- What is actually being said versus what you would normally expect to be said
- What isn't said (e.g., attempts to evade a question)
- When something is said (e.g., statement out of the blue)
- How something is said (e.g., changes in loudness, pitch, or rate of speech)
- Unnatural pauses
- Sudden changes of topic
- Times the person suddenly becomes silent or talkative
- What the person does and doesn't respond to

- Reactions to your remarks
- Sudden changes in posture or body position
- Times when the person looks down or away
- Times when the person acts distant or defensive
- Times when the person looks more steadily and intently at you, or through you rather than at you
- Changes in facial expression (e.g., sudden smiles or frowns)
- Restless movement, or motionlessness
- Sudden changes in mood (e.g., relaxation to anxiety, or vice versa)
- Sudden increases or decreases in interest

Reading between the lines is especially important when you are dealing with a dying person. Dying people frequently sense when they are dying, even if their friends and family may see no indications of it. Those who are dying often use the metaphor of travel to alert those around that it is time for them to die.

Frequently the dying try to share information about their dying by using symbolic language. They tell stories, discuss their dreams, talk about another place, and see or hold conversations with people who are invisible to others present. Dying people want very much for these happenings to be understood. It is important to them that they express their inner longings, but regrettably they often encounter difficulty, whether in expressing these thoughts or in getting them understood.

To understand a critically ill person's symbolic messages, you must listen carefully, listening between the lines. But listening between the lines is difficult; it requires tremendous desire and an all-out effort on your part. Fortunately, however, the understanding you gain is well worth the effort.

35

Listening to the Whole Person

So when you are listening to somebody, completely, attentively, then you are listening not only to the words, but also to the feelings being conveyed, to the whole of it, not part of it.
—J. Krishnamurti

Most people want desperately to be listened to. Ill people, in particular, have a deep, unending need to be heard and understood. Perhaps the first duty of love is to truly listen to a loved one—and it is important as well to show that you are listening, and that you have heard. Listening is an acknowledgment of caring. Ask yourself: "Do I listen to others in the way I would like to be listened to?"

Hearing and listening are not the same thing. Hearing is a physical process that occurs naturally, and without effort. Listening, however, is a mental process that requires definite effort. Effective listening is a demanding task that requires hard work and commitment.

Listening has two stages:
1. Hearing what is said
2. Responding to what is heard

There can be no effective listening without an appropriate response, whether it be verbal or nonverbal. Listening involves both attitude and technique; it is a complicated process involving much more than looking attentively and hearing what was said.

The greatest reward of being a good listener is knowing that by listening well you are genuinely helping someone who is ill. Conversely, bad listening can devastate a sick person who is saying something he or she considers important (or personal). Feeling ignored or misunderstood can make an ill person want to withdraw into feelings of loneliness and futility.

Often, sick people want you to simply listen to them, rather than to give them advice or solve their problems. They want only for you to stop talking, to really listen to them in a compassionate, nonjudgmental manner. Typically, the way you listen to someone determines how freely and honestly a sick person will talk with you.

To be an effective listener, you must listen totally, to the entire person. Use your eyes, ears, body position, brain, and heart, as well as all your senses. Listening to the total person means you listen to his or her words, tone of voice, and body language.

Listening effectively to a sick person requires that you convey that you are always available to listen to him or her. Being truly available means that you are both physically accessible and mentally approachable. When a friend or family member has a long-term illness, even though you are genuinely committed to being available to helping the person, you may experience some physical and emotional burnout (see Appendix A for symptoms). This is natural; you shouldn't feel guilty, or feel that you have let the ill person down. We all have limited strength and energy— we can only do so much, and no more.

By being aware of some common obstacles to effective listening, you will be better able to avoid them:

- Being and acting preoccupied
- Making quick judgments, and jumping to conclusions
- Being inattentive, and listening intermittently
- Being distracted, and thinking of other things you have to do
- Sitting uncomfortably, or sitting at different heights
- Assuming you understand something when you don't
- Interrupting, or abruptly changing the subject
- Listening to refute, rather than to understand
- Thinking about what you are going to say next
- Focusing on facts, and ignoring the feelings expressed
- Failing to try to understand what is said from the viewpoint of the person saying it

Another major barrier to effective listening is that most of us have no idea of just how poor listeners we really are. Few of us have any training in how to be a good listener. But fortunately, you can train yourself to be an effective listener. Each of us has the ability to improve our listening skills.

Begin improving your listening skills by wanting to listen. Next, monitor your listening habits to identify the bad habits you need to eliminate. (It is best to work on only a few bad habits at a time.) Finally, conscientiously practice recommended techniques for listening. Improving your listening abilities is largely a matter of attitude. Admittedly, it requires considerable effort, but the effort pays off.

Your listening style reflects your attitude and behavior as a listener. Strive to be an active listener. You can't be a lazy listener and still be a good listener. An active listener tries to understand what the person who is talking is actually thinking and feeling, as well as what the message being sent really means. An active listener must want to hear what the person speaking has to say, and must be willing to take the time to hear the person out. The active listener does not send concurrent messages of his or her own. Instead, he or she restricts his or her responses to what the speaker has said. Appropriate responses include relevant statements, clarifying questions, and, sometimes, interested silence.

The active listener seeks to verify that he or she understands what has been said by putting what was said into his or her own words, and by asking questions about what was heard. An active listener accepts his or her own feelings and allows the other person to have his or her own feelings and perceptions about things. The active listener listens to the feelings expressed compassionately and the facts expressed objectively. And, most important of all, the active listener desires to be a good listener and is willing to work hard to improve his or her listening abilities.

Effective listeners use the following recommended techniques for listening to ill people:

- Wants to listen, and shows it
- Puts the speaker at ease, helping him or her feel comfortable
- Makes himself or herself comfortable in order to give full attention to what is said
- Sits down to show that "I'm here and have time to listen to you"
- Looks, and acts, interested, sitting alertly with his or her eyes centered on the speaker
- Sits nearby and leans forward, nodding frequently and responding by appropriate facial expressions
- Absorbs all that is said—acts like a sponge
- Encourages the speaker to say what is on his or her mind, to express his or her feelings—and then acknowledges these feelings in a manner that shows understanding (e.g., by repeating a couple of key words to show evidence of listening and understanding)
- Gives appropriate responses
- Asks relevant questions about what was said, without intimidating the person speaking
- Empathizes with the ill person by putting himself or herself in his or her position

- Gets rid of distractions
- Tailors listening style to adapt to the person speaking while looking and acting natural
- Looks for body language clues to enhance understanding
- Gives supportive feedback, such as, "I see what you mean," "I hear you," nodding accompanied by an *uh huh* sound

Few of us are good listeners, but thankfully we can all become skillful listeners if we want to, and if we practice recommended ways to listen effectively.

36

Listening When It Counts

Sometimes it is a great joy just to listen to someone we love talking with.

—Vincent McNabb

As a rule, it is best to listen to an ill person any time he or she wants to talk. However, there are times when it is especially important to listen:

- When the person is experiencing pain
- When the person has had an especially rough day
- When the person is feeling lonely and depressed
- When the person is frightened
- When the person has just received bad news
- When the person has just been informed of a new diagnosis
- When person is expressing regret over being a burden
- When the person's body language indicates a need for it
- When the person is facing death

However, possible exceptions to the rule of always listening, based on the particular situation and on circumstances—though rare—could presumably include

- When the person is acting extremely abusively toward you
- When you feel you are losing your self-control and need time to regain your composure
- When the person is acting irrational or incoherent under the effects of medication
- When the person needs to be quiet and conserve his or her energy at a critical time
- When the person has expressed a desire to be alone and doesn't want to talk anymore

But remember: it is prudent to listen at all times except when there are definite legitimate reasons for not doing so for a certain time.

PART 4

RELATING

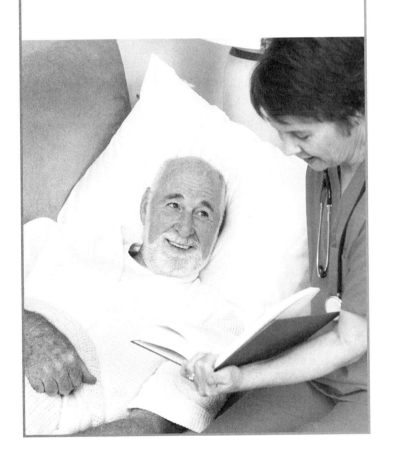

37

Being Humorous

*Humor is a serious thing. I like to think of it
as one of our greatest and earliest natural resources
that must be preserved at all costs.*
—James Thurber

Laughter and humor are important aspects of life. To be humorous is to be human in the finest sense. Chronic illness is certainly not a laughing matter, but the chronically ill need to laugh, and laugh often. Good-natured teasing, kidding around, and laughing together are big equalizers between those who are well and those who are sick. Shared laughter creates a feeling of togetherness. Your humor helps cheer up sick people and makes them look forward to being with you.

Humor is one of our greatest human assets, because it helps relieve stress, and sometimes even pain. Laughter contributes to overall good health. Humor is an important coping mechanism that also improves the quality of life of those who are ill. Laughter is healing—it makes all people feel better.

So how does laughter improve a person's health? In many ways: An individual's diaphragm, thorax, abdomen, heart, lungs, and even liver are massaged during a hearty laugh. What's more, brain researchers suspect that laughter activates the release of endorphins—the body's own pain-relieving substance. Since laughter helps the body provide its own medicine, try to be alert to opportunities to inject humor when interacting with ill folks.

Your personality influences how effective you are in using humor to cheer up an ill person. You aren't expected to be a comedian, but you probably already have the ability to be humorous. You don't have to be a professional entertainer to be entertaining and to provoke laughter. And best of all, humor is a learnable skill. Becoming humorous begins with a desire to be.

Tailor your humor to the individual—in particular, be sure in every instance to make your humor socially acceptable. Tease only in the right ways, and never to excess. Avoid being obscene. And it's a good idea to size up the ill person's mood, and how he or she is feeling, before saying anything humorous. In some cases, a hearty laugh may make pain worse. In such cases, positive intent can have a negative result.

Realize that humor can't be imposed on someone else. A humorless person, for example, may resent your use of humor. So watch the person's reactions to your humor. If the response is negative, stop immediately, and wait until he or she seems to be in a more receptive mood—perhaps until after he or she has said something humorous. Also, recognize that what some people consider humorous may appear to be anything but to others. So be flexible—and sensitive.

Being able to laugh at ourselves and our predicaments endears us to our friends and family. The most humorous stories and anecdotes are those in which we are personally involved. Reciting your mishaps, misdeeds, and so on in a self-deprecating way can delight the person you're talking with. Look for chances to laugh at yourself, and others will laugh with you; we all need to be able to laugh at ourselves to enjoy life as fully as possible. And try to tell stories and anecdotes that are short and easy to follow; an ill person may lack the energy or attention span to comprehend long, involved accounts.

As we all know, a joke can evoke hilarious laughter . . . or it may fall completely flat. Few people tell jokes well. Unless you are really good at telling jokes, it is probably best not to tell them at all; even professional comedians sometimes have a hard time making people laugh. And if you do tell a joke, avoid touchy topics so you don't risk causing offense. Ethnic jokes or jokes of a sexual nature can blow up in your face, because by their nature they can degrade people; consequently, many people object to them.

There are other problems to be aware of when telling jokes to a sick person. Jokes are artificial humor—they are not spontaneous and are designed to provoke laughter. You can't predict reactions to your jokes. Perhaps more importantly, hearing a joke puts pressure on the person listening to laugh. In a sense hearing a joke creates an obligation to respond with laughter whether genuine or faked. Note also that if an ill person tells a joke it may be a false signal. It may be an attempt to be brave when the person really feels bad or vulnerable.

A caution about teasing. Teasing can be mutually enjoyable or it can be irritating and cause resentment. All teasing should be well intended and never malicious. Teasing takes place when you use a little bit of aggression to show your affection for a person. However, when teasing an ill person you need to be super careful not to put down the person or be perceived as insulting. Teasing can also be done to excess so you need to know when to stop.

Here are several tips regarding the use of humor with ill people:

- Tell—better yet, share—humorous stories and anecdotes.
- Be alert to appropriate opportunities to share humor.
- Introduce the element of surprise with your humor.
- Smile and chuckle moderately—don't get carried away by your own funniness.
- Let your humor arise naturally from the situation, rather than contriving it.
- Keep on the lookout for humorous events and jokes to share—write them down so you can remember them.

- Speak clearly and loudly enough to be heard easily—don't mutter or drop your voice at the end of sentences.
- Limit the amount of humor you share at one time.
- Be brief and to the point—don't overwhelm the person with details.
- Avoid being so subtle that the person doesn't get the humor you have to share.
- Speak at a measured rate—don't rush.
- Pause at the right times to build up suspense.
- On occasion, give the person joke books, humorous tapes, and funny videos instead of flowers and candy to spice up gift-giving.

Humor is one of your greatest assets for creating and maintaining harmonious relationships with ill people. And it can be healing; laughter is good for the soul. This quotation from John Billings is worth remembering: "There ain't much fun in medicine, but there is a heck of a lot of medicine in fun."

38

Being Perceptive

Men quite gladly believe what they want to believe.
—Ovid

You can't expect other people to perceive or view things the same way you do. Why? Because we are all unique and different. We all perceive and react to things differently. In a sense, we all live in different worlds. We tend to see what we want to see, to hear what we want to hear, and to remember what we want to remember. We filter what is said or done to us based on our own reality, according to the way we view the world.

The way you are perceived by an ill person is crucial to your relationship with him or her. The perceived "you" is just as important to the relationship as the real you is. In essence, you are who an ill person perceives you to be.

A chronically ill person's reactions to you aren't necessarily related to something you have said or done. His or her reaction may be based on his or her own past experience with a person you remind him or her of. (For example, the author was once unable to establish good rapport with a female co-worker, despite his best efforts,

because he strongly resembled someone who had left
her at the altar. She, bitter about such horrible treatment,
consequently tried to avoid the author as much as possible.)

A person's response to what you say and do is strongly
influenced by his or her perception of you. An oft-quoted
statement in communications circles makes this point
powerfully: "How can I hear what you are saying when
there is so much of you saying it?"

Perceptions are frequently inexact and distorted. For
example, you may be trying your best to be helpful to an ill
person, but your actions may be resented because they are
perceived as being intrusive and controlling.

Perceptions are very personal and often have meaning
only to the person perceiving the situation or event. For
example, sometimes a seriously ill appears to be reaching
for someone or responding to somebody utterly beyond
your own perception, even though you are in the same
room together.

You must achieve a common perception of things
with a sick person if you are going to be able to truly share
experiences. An amusing story illustrates how a lack of
mutual perception can cause misunderstandings: One
evening a nurse in the surgery ward of a hospital noticed
that a patient who was scheduled for a routine operation
early the next morning had not eaten his dinner. She also
noticed that an orderly had begun collecting dinner trays
in nearby rooms. Not wanting the patient to go hungry,
the nurse said tersely, "You had better hurry up and eat
while you still can." This stern statement alarmed the

patient greatly; he interpreted the statement as an indication that he must be much sicker than he had been led to believe, and that the surgery must be life-threatening. Just as in this story, sometimes those who are ill are inclined to read in things that aren't really said or done. Because of this, you must be sensitive to how even your most innocent statements can be misinterpreted.

You and someone who is ill are going to disagree on things from time to time, simply because of your differing perceptions. It is important to recognize that when you and an ill person disagree on an issue, he or she thinks he or she is just as right as you believe you are. And he or she is just as eager for you to accept his or her viewpoint on the matter as you may want him or her to accept yours.

It is equally important to realize that a person's perceptions change very slowly and gradually—if at all. For example, if an ill person initially dislikes his or her doctor, this feeling is likely to persist. In fact, an ill person, in most instances, is not likely to exert the energy required to reassess his or her perceptions of people or events.

We usually don't question the accuracy of our own perceptions; after all, we saw it with our own eyes and heard it with our own ears, so that must be the way it really is. Nevertheless, it is essential that you try to view things as the ill person views them, in order to gain mutual understanding. The more closely you can perceive the sick person as he or she actually is, the better you will relate to him or her.

It is imperative that you

- Get feedback to check out the accuracy of your own perceptions on important matters (e.g., "What do you think I meant when I said . . .")
- Give feedback to check out the accuracy of your perceptions on important matters (e.g., "As I understand it, you want me to . . .")

The more frequently you check the accuracy of your perceptions, the better. Verifying your perception on important matters is absolutely essential.

The way you are perceived by an ill person largely influences how well you relate with each other. The best way to discern how you are perceived as a person is to observe the ill person's attitude and behavior toward you, as carefully and objectively as possible.

A simple way to check out your perception of something an ill person has said is to rephrase what you think you heard to be sure you understand it correctly. Conversely, to verify that an ill person has heard you the way you intended to be heard, ask him or her to tell you, in his or her own words, what he or she understood you to say.

An understanding of the basic principles of perception will help you understand and be understood better when talking with an ill friend or loved one. Also, remember to verify that you understand what a person has said—and, in turn, to confirm that have been understood—when discussing anything important.

39

Being Supportive

You can stroke people with words.
—F. Scott Fitzgerald

Chronically ill people need your supportive statements—so make supportive comments whenever you can. However, realize that you need to tailor your comments to the sick individual's personality and the particular situation. This means that you need to pick and choose your comments, rather than assuming that a certain recommended statement can be used to fit all ill people and all occasions (one size does *not* fit all).

When you make a supportive statement or response, you show that you care for the person, and that you have a "warm, fuzzy feeling" about him or her. Supporting an ill person means that you back up and uphold what he or she says and does whenever you can. But you can't do this carte blanche—for example, when he or she makes foolish decisions or requests that would be detrimental to his or her health. When you are supportive, you help and comfort someone. In addition, it means you defend a position he or she takes on an issue, when it makes sense to do so; take, for example, his or her refusal to take a new medicine that may cause him or her to feel drowsy, or sick to his or her stomach.

Although we will be primarily focusing on supportive statements at this time, it is important to note that you can show your support without saying anything. For example, you can make reassuring sounds, such as *hmm* and *ahh* at appropriate times as a response. Your facial expressions can also indicate your support—for example, nodding, direct eye contact, and frequent smiling.

Let's explore various statements you may elect to use:

Presence and Availability

- "I'm here for you whenever you need me."
- "You're on my mind constantly; I'm always available to help you."
- "You took care of me when I needed you, and now I'm honored to have the opportunity to reciprocate."
- "I want to assure you that I want to be with you as much as I possibly can—I don't see it merely as a duty."
- "I feel honored to be around you. You can count on me being here for you."

Desire to Help

- "I am ready to help you in any way I can—I just need you to tell me how I can best help you."

- "I don't know if you need my help, but I really want to help out, if you want me to."
- "Yesterday, you mentioned that you would like your room rearranged. Would you like me to help you with it?"
- "I understand your wanting to do as much on your own as you possibly can, but if you would like my help on anything, I'd love to help you."
- "I wish I knew of more ways to help you be more comfortable, but I'm stumped—let me know if you think of anything that we can do to help."
- "It really makes me feel good when I can do things to help you."

Being Around the Person
- "I really look forward to talking with you."
- "Being with you means a lot to me."
- "I love it when we do things together."
- "I want you to know how much I love you and enjoy being with you."
- "My visits with you are the highlight of my day."
- "I miss being with you when I have to be out of town."
- "Having you involved in family activities makes them more enjoyable."

Understanding the Person
- "I understand."
- "I hear what you're saying."

- "I know what you mean."
- "Yep, I've been there too."
- "I bet I'd feel exactly the same way if I were in your position."
- "It's obvious this matter is very important to you."
- "I share your concerns about the new nurse."
- "That certainly must be frustrating for you."
- "I can tell that you're in great pain."
- "As I understand it, you feel that you should . . ."
- "That must really upset you."
- "I share your sorrow about that."

Making the Person Feel Important

- "I would like to hear your suggestions for . . ."
- "I need your advice on something, if I may."
- "I would like to know your ideas for . . ."
- "I want to check this out with you before I decide to . . ."
- "I would appreciate your opinion on . . ."
- "We don't know what to do, and we could use your input to help us decide what to do."
- "I trust your judgment on this matter."
- "Because you know better than I . . ."
- "What is your gut feeling about what we should do?"

Desire to Listen

- "Tell me more about how it feels to be . . ."
- "I like listening to your stories about . . ."

- "I can't wait to hear what you think about . . ."
- "I'm here to listen to anything that concerns you."
- "Listening to you is a real treat for me."
- "I'm willing to listen to anything you want to talk about."
- "I find everything you say interesting."

Making Decisions and Solving Problems

- "Let's work on the problem together—I'm sure we can figure out a solution."
- "Whatever you decide will be fine with me."
- "I think you've identified all the possible solutions to the problem; do you want to discuss them together?"
- "I think you're in a better position to decide that than I am."
- "If you want my help in making a decision on that, I'll help you any way I can."

The Person's Health Condition

- "I feel for you—it must be tough bearing so much pain."
- "I'm pleased to see you getting around so well."
- "Your voice sounds stronger today!"
- "You have more color than the last time I saw you."
- "I hear you got out of bed yesterday and walked around—that's great!"
- "I'm told that your exercises went well yesterday—keep up the good work!"

- "Your nurse says you're eating better—that's great news!"
- "You may be feeling weak, but your mind is as sharp as ever."
- "I like to see you laugh so much."
- "Tell me more about how you feel."
- "It sounds as though you are feeling . . ."
- "It is difficult for me to imagine what you are going through, but I know it isn't easy."
- "I share your concern about the seriousness of your illness."

It is equally important to make supportive responses to what an ill person tells you whenever it is feasible to do so. Your responses are supportive when you show that you understand the feelings an ill person expresses.

These two examples should be helpful:

1. If the ill person says, "I keep having painful headaches," you could respond, "I'm sorry you're having such painful headaches. I can't do anything to help you myself, but I'll call your doctor immediately if you'd like me to."

2. If the ill person says, "I am feeling lonely and isolated," you could reply, "I'm sorry you're feeling so lonely. That must be terrible. But I'm here with you now, and I'm willing to be here any time you need me." You might also want to add, "Is there anyone in particular you want to see so I can let them know?"

These two examples should give you an idea of the many kinds of supportive statements you could make when the need arises.

It is worth keeping the following points in mind whenever you make supportive comments:

- Statements giving premature assurance (before the facts are known) don't really reassure, and they may offer false hope.
- Judgmental statements tend to retard, and even end, conversations.
- Your responses have a strong impact on the future direction of a conversation.
- Despite your desire to be supportive, you can't expect to effectively respond to all requests, or to agree with everything the ill person says or does.

40

Being Tactful

Diplomacy is to do and say the nastiest things
in the nicest way.
—ISAAC GOLDBERG

Chronically ill people appreciate being spoken to in a tactful manner. To be tactful, take the time to think before saying anything. Try to word the things you say as politely and diplomatically as possible, especially if you are going to say something negative or critical. It is both uncaring and unwise to blurt out the first thing that comes to your mind regardless of the consequences. The purpose of your being with the ill person is to maintain good will, and to comfort the person. Speaking bluntly and acting abrasively not only defeats this purpose, but can trigger resentment and ill will.

Being tactful includes
- Being thoughtful and considerate
- Possessing a keen sense of what to say and do
- Acting graciously and diplomatically
- Saying only what is proper and in good taste

- Being sensitive to other people's feelings and needs
- Being discrete in all you say and do
- Handling touchy situations delicately, and with finesse
- Avoiding unnecessary confrontation

Granted—it is sometimes challenging, if not downright difficult, to be candid and tactful at the same time. Nevertheless, you must constantly strive to say the right things, using the right words, in the right way; otherwise, you risk offending the sick person. Being tactful also involves knowing when it is best to be noncommittal. If your gut urges you to say something that won't do any good, and that may even hurt the sick person's feelings, it is better to remain silent.

Here are several things you can do to be tactful:

- Disagree without being disagreeable.
- Use the term *difference of opinion* instead of *disagreement* when you and the ill person view things differently. This simple change in terminology is less emotionally charged, and incites less heat.
- Object without being objectionable. Differ calmly without raising your voice. To avoid being offensive, ask questions rather than making bold statements: "Don't you think the time has come to begin using a feeding tube so you will feel stronger?" This approach is far better than saying, "I strongly believe the time has come to begin using a feeding tube, since you're having so much trouble eating."

- Make requests instead of demands: "Would you please finish your meal so you can take your nap?" is more tactful than saying, "I want you to finish your meal right now; it's past time for you to take your nap."

- Use euphemisms (judiciously) rather than harsh graphic words: "Your lack of exercise is making you look heavier lately," is preferable to saying, "Your failure to exercise properly is making you look fat." Also, try to use inoffensive expressions: "I think your skipping meals is making you appear quite thin," is better than the abrasive "Your stubborn refusal to eat right is making you look emaciated."

When you use euphemisms and inoffensive statements to avoid offending sick people, be careful not to say things so indirectly and gently that the person listening misses the point you are trying to make. Your challenge is to find the right balance between tact and honesty.

- Avoid correcting something insignificant that an ill person says. In particular, it is a cardinal sin to bluntly contradict him or her. What difference does it make—how does it help anything—to correct a wrong date, a person's name, or some other irrelevant detail? When these "mistakes" happen, simply overlook them and say nothing.

- Talk about people you both know in positive, rather than negative, terms: "Uncle Jack hasn't been able

to visit you much as he would like to lately, because
he has been so busy at work," is certainly better
than saying, "You know how Uncle Jack is—he's so
preoccupied with his own activities that he has little
time for anyone else." When you speak disparagingly
about the ill person's friends or family members, it
doesn't help anything, and it could prove harmful.

Politeness and tact are free, and they really pay off
in improved relationships. You can never go wrong by
routinely saying *please*, *thank you*, and *you're welcome*.
Remembering the "little things" and niceties is an
important part of tact.

41

Developing Rapport

Treat people as they want to be treated,
not as you want to be treated.
—Walt St. John

You develop rapport with an ill person when you have the right attitude, say and do the right things at the right time and in the right way.

To create rapport, you need to be genuinely helpful, and to be viewed as such by the ailing person. It is essential that you know when help is helpful, and when it is harmful. For example, it is not to do something for a person who wants, and is able, to do the it himself or herself. An ill individual needs to know you are available and can be relied upon to help him when needed.

You need to be an other-centered person to establish rapport. You need to send the clear message that the ill person, not yourself, is your primary concern. To do this, stress *you* in your conversations, and deemphasize *I*. Show the ill person that you like, respect, accept, and value him or her. Demonstrate that you view him or her as an equal; never act superior or condescending in any way.

You promote rapport when you act natural and have the courage to be who you really are. Be real. Be genuine. Be yourself. Don't put on an act for the sick person's benefit, and don't mask your real feelings.

Build trust by being predictable and acting consistently. Show the person that you trust him or her, and that you can be trusted. This is vital, because trust is the cornerstone to all close and enduring relationships. You build trust by letting the ill person know what he or she can expect from you, by honoring your promises, and by following up on his or her requests. In addition, sharing and honoring confidences fosters trust.

Help the ailing person feel safe and comfortable around you by unconditionally accepting him or her as he or she is and dealing with him or her in a nonjudgmental manner. By creating a feeling of mutual involvement and having common interests, you further build rapport. Emphasizing your similarities and downplaying your differences creates rapport. By avoiding unnecessary confrontation, you can prevent conflict and hard feelings. Whenever you disagree, try to do so agreeably.

It is a serious mistake to focus excessively on a person's illness; by doing so, you risk replacing the rest of the person's identity. It is important to realize that a person's illness is only a small part of the person; there is a lot of the person remaining. The loss of identity as a complete person with value and worth may be strongly resented by the ill person, whose needs for a full identity are the same as those of the well people around him or her.

Chronically ill people continue to need to feel important, to have dignity, to be respected, and to be involved in matters affecting them and their families. They want to be treated as somebodies, to be appreciated and approved of regardless of their medical condition. They need to control their life and activities as much as possible, and not to have their responsibilities taken over by others—they want to live while they are alive.

Try your best not to strip the ailing person of his or her dignity and feeling of being valued. By saying and doing the following things, you can promote an ill individual's feelings of value and worth:

- Let the person control his or her life and be responsible for himself or herself as much as his or her condition, and the situation, permit.
- Avoid showing any signs that you feel pity for the person.
- Refrain from trying to change the person or his or her surroundings to suit your own desires.
- Treat him or her as an equal.
- Use adult language, and talk adult-to-adult, not as parent-to-child.
- Show the person respect, and be certain that he or she knows you respect him or her.
- Resist the temptation to be overly solicitous and helpful.
- Help him or her to feel needed, wanted, and loved.
- Look for ways to give earned praise.

- Treat him or her as a complete individual, rather than as a stereotype or a case.

Having and demonstrating the right attitude will help you to have harmonious relationships with ill people. By doing the following, you can show the right attitude:

- Greet the person warmly, and with a big smile.
- Be natural, and act relaxed.
- Desire to be genuinely helpful, as needed and as wanted.
- Act enthusiastic and pleased to be with the person, rather than as if you're just doing your duty.

To talk meaningfully with an ill person, you first must show that you trust and respect him or her. It's important to talk in terms of the other person's interests, but try not to talk too much about his or her health problems. Show a sincere interest in what he or she has to say rather than simply listening in order to be polite. Know when it is best for you to talk, and when it is best to remain silent.

Try to avoid saying things that will upset a sick person. When you are compelled to say something that you know will displease the person, say it gently and tactfully. It is best to avoid making judgmental statements—they generally irritate people.

You further enhance dialogue when you talk in a quiet, private, comfortable setting. Make sure the type of and the placement of the bed, chairs, and other furniture suits the needs and tastes of the ill person, rather than yours. If the ill person is satisfied with the furniture and furnishings the way they are, let them alone. Don't touch anything. This permissive approach lets the ill person know that he or she is still in control of things, and that his or her opinion is the one that counts. Try to stand or sit close enough to the person so you can touch him or her at appropriate times in appropriate ways.

Finally, you encourage relaxed and candid conversation when you create a permissive climate that enables the chronically ill person to feel free to express his or her opinions, beliefs, and innermost feelings. Also, by injecting humor at appropriate times, you help loosen things up.

Remember the importance of "the little things"—getting the person a glass of water, rearranging the pillows, sitting at the same level so you can see each other easily, engaging in small talk, and so forth. By paying attention to the little things, you help the person feel important and comfortable in your presence.

Rapport is reinforced when you are supportive and responsive, especially in tough times for the ill person, such as

- A change for the worse in the person's health condition
- The impending approach of something very important of a negative nature
- Bad news that needs to be conveyed

Remember these points when trying to build the ill person's self-esteem and feelings of worth:

- They matter because they are.
- Say thank you for being you.
- Everyone wants to feel like, and be treated as, a somebody.

42

Developing Trust

Trust, like the soul, never returns, once it is gone.
—Publilius Syrus

We all have an intense need to trust and to be trusted. This is a universal truth, a part of the human condition.

You must show your trust if someone else is to trust you. Trust is reciprocal thing: trust begets trust. Building trust is required before any meaningful relationship can be established with a chronically ill person. Candid, honest communication requires trust—unless an ailing person trusts you, he or she will not risk sharing important thoughts and feelings with you.

There are many things you can do to develop trust:

- Reveal something highly personal and sensitive about yourself.
- Keep your promises—and don't promise something you can't produce.
- Follow up on legitimate requests within a reasonable time.

- Protect and honor all confidences shared with you.
- Be genuinely helpful and nonmanipulative.
- Have a reputation as a person of principle and integrity.
- Accept your responsibilities, and act in a responsible manner.
- Be fair, acting ethically in all your dealings with others.
- Be sincere, candid, and truthful in all you say.
- Be available when needed.
- Act predictably and consistently.
- Be certain your actions match your words.
- Speak and act confidently.
- Hear people out, and don't jump to conclusions.
- Show the ill person that you believe in his or her ability to make decisions and to accept responsibility for and take control of his or her life (as much as his or her condition permits).
- Show that you accept, respect, and understand the person.
- Let the sick person know up front what he or she can and can't expect from you, and act accordingly.
- Make sure your tone of voice, your words, and your body language all send the same messages, especially when discussing important matters.
- Be willing to say, "I don't know," rather than guessing or bluffing when you answer an ill person's questions.

Realize that building trust takes time. If you do something to lose a person's trust, it will be hard to regain—sometimes it may be impossible to regain fully. As the saying goes, "People may forgive, but they never forget." So do your best to maintain your credibility, and try never to do anything to jeopardize it.

43

Having a Proper Attitude

A merry heart doeth good like a medicine.
—Proverbs 17:22

A proper attitude is the foundation of your relationship
with an ill person. Your attitude determines how you
look, what you say, and how you act around a friend or
loved one who is ailing.

You need to convey immediately that you care for the
person, that you are truly available, and that you want
to help in any way possible. Show the person that you
consider him or her to be important and highly valued,
somebody who is special to you.

Talk to the person in a kind manner—and as an equal.
Don't act controlling, superior, or condescending. Make
your attitude shout, "I'm okay, and you're okay—we're both
okay!" Emphasize that both of you count.

Make yourself someone who is easy to be around by
always putting the sick person first. Give his or her needs
first priority in all that you say and do. When you greet
the person, exude an attitude of, "there you are," not "here

I am." Treat the ill person as he or she wants to be treated, not as you want to be treated: you are two different people, with different needs, wants, ways of thinking, and ways of doing things.

Even though your attitude should be other-centered, you must realize that you, too, have needs and feelings that you must acknowledge, and that you must deal with. Know in advance how emotionally involved you are willing to be with the sick person. If you decide to make a full commitment, remember that—empathetic as you may feel—the sick person must own his or her own problems. It is unwise for you to take over his or her problems and make them your own.

It is wise to act natural and be honest with an ill person. You need to be compassionate about the person and his or her problems, but be objective about his or her physical condition and future prospects. Be happy, and feel honored to be with your sick friend or relative. Be calm and relaxed—transmit a reassuring, soothing presence. And be comfortable to be with; recognize that forced optimism and cheerfulness are transparent, and may inhibit the honest expression of feelings by both of you.

Your attitude should be positive, yet realistic. It is ill-advised (and dishonest) to express false hope, but on the other hand, it is best not to project feelings of frustration and futility about the person's condition and future. Refrain from acting sad and angry over the situation. Be patient, and make the best of things. Try not to act moody or depressed when around a person who is sick, because this makes matters worse for all concerned.

Show a willingness to share information openly, in a sincere, straightforward manner. Be willing to level with the person, telling him or he what he or she wants to know rather than only what you want to tell. Share some personal information about yourself to encourage the sick person to reciprocate—and when he or she does, prove that you understand what you have been told. When discussing personal and sensitive private matters, show that you can be trusted by protecting all confidential information. Try to learn the "little things" that matter to the person to promote a feeling of togetherness and intimacy. For example, find out his or her nickname, pet peeves, interests, favorite colors, and so on.

Be willing to be primarily a listener, and to be responsive to what you hear. Discipline yourself to hear the person out, and to listen to understand rather than merely to be polite or to refute what has been said. Be patient, and listen carefully to what is being said, even though it may be rambling and difficult to follow. Encourage the person to share life stories to build his or her spirits, and to create bridges of mutual understanding.

But be careful not to make unwarranted assumptions. It's a mistake to confuse physical infirmities with mental deterioration. Have—and convey—a deep, sincere respect for the person, and for his or her need to maintain control of his or her own life.

And keep a flexible attitude, allowing yourself to quickly adjust to an ill person's changing moods, needs, and physical condition.

44

Having Realistic Expectations

*The quality of our expectations
determines the quality of our action.*
—André Godin

It is wise not to have any specific expectations for dealing with a chronically ill person. Expect that each person and each situation will be different, and will need to be treated differently. What you can know for sure is that you will need an open mind, and that you will need to be flexible. You need to be able to adapt quickly to the ill person's changing needs, moods, and health condition. The ill person will have his or her ups and downs, as well as his or her good days and bad days—so you can take things only one day at a time.

You can also expect to pay an emotional price for your involvement. You may need to witness pain, juggle competing demands on your time, be the brunt of anger, and even face approaching death with the person. Expect normal family relationships and routines to be disturbed; for example, the roles of parents and children may be reversed. The whole family is affected when a family member becomes chronically ill. Caring for an ill family member is not just hard work, but an all-consuming matter that affects all aspects of life.

Try to be as helpful as you possibly can, but don't expect too much from yourself. You can only do your best—no more. You can't always be available. You can't know everything about the person's illness, or how to make him or her pain-free and comfortable all the time. You can't expect to have answers to all the questions you are asked. You can't be and do everything for the ill person. At times, you will be taxed to your limits; it is essential that you realize that you have limited time, energy, and ability, and that you yourself will need help sometimes.

Don't expect to feel relaxed, patient, and upbeat all the time when you have the responsibility of caring for a sick friend or loved one. Regrettably, despite your good intentions and heroic efforts, you probably won't receive many expressions of gratitude and appreciation for your help. Most people tend to take others for granted and simply fail to show their appreciation for things done for them. Thus, you can expect to feel unappreciated and disheartened at times—perhaps even used. At worst, you may be insulted, criticized, and even resented (many people resent being dependent on others). In such cases, you must be accepting and unendingly patient.

Expect that it will take time to gain the trust of, and form a close bond with, a person who becomes ill. Don't feel discouraged, or feel that you have done something wrong, if this doesn't occur immediately. You will also need to balance your desire to be positive and hopeful about the person's condition with the harsh reality of the situation. This is not easy.

Expect to be required to adapt at any given moment to the ill person's changing moods and unpredictable behavior. At times, the person may be serious or lighthearted, mentally alert or sluggish, in pain or pain-free, apathetic or lively, and so on. In these changing situations, you must be able to go with the flow, adjusting your type of help to the particular situation.

Sometimes the ill person will be eager to have you present; at other times, he or she may prefer to be alone. Sometimes he or she will want to talk excessively; at others, he or she will fall silent. He or she may want to talk seriously, in a no-nonsense manner, sometimes, and at other times, to joke around and engage in small talk. Sometimes he or she will show great interest in the national and world scene; at others, he or she will show no interest in anything other than the events of his or her own life.

Many ill people like to talk more than to listen. They have more of a desire to be understood by you than to understand you. At times, an ill person will refuse to talk about his or her physical ailments; at others he or she will talk nonstop about them.

Expect some conflict between an ill person's desire for independence and his or her need to be dependent. Try not to take control and be overly protective, but accept that you may need to exert certain controls because of the demands of the situation. Whenever you do need to act controlling, you can usually expect the person to be resistant and resentful; most people like to control their own lives. In order to minimize negative reaction, try to involve the person as much as possible in decisions that affect him or her.

Because you are only human, expect to have ambivalent feelings about the constant need to care for an ill person—no matter how much you love the individual. You don't need to feel guilty when you have these mixed feelings, because you continue to have your own needs, issues, and problems to deal with.

You may—understandably—feel overwhelmed by your responsibilities and by the competing demands on your time. You may want to shout, "Hey, I'm only one person—take it easy on me!" But try not to play the "woe is me" or "ain't it awful" games. You may also feel some misapprehension about an uncertain and unpredictable future, since the unknown frustrates and frightens all of us.

Expect a chronically ill, especially critically ill person, to put you on the spot occasionally with questions about his or her condition and future. He or she will expect answers even when it may be impossible or inappropriate for you to provide them. The best way for you to respond to these kinds of questions is to explain in a caring way that you can't answer the questions; for example, you might say, "I'm sorry, but I don't have a crystal ball—I'm not any more sure about the future than you are."

You can expect that sometimes dying people may confuse you by reciting strange dreams or by talking to someone in the room who is invisible to you. Rather than merely dismissing these dreams and encounters as pure fantasy, accept that their occurrence is important, and real, to the dying person.

In instances like these, it is prudent to ask the dying person to tell you more about the dreams and the invisible people with whom he or she is talking with. Such conversations can be enjoyable for the dying person, and informative to you.

There are also many positive experiences you can expect to have when caring for an ill friend or loved one, including

- Many enjoyable and interesting conversations
- Joy and pleasure from genuinely helping someone
- The opportunity to bond and form a closer relationship
- Feelings of honor springing from association on such an intimate basis
- An opportunity for self-growth by service to others
- Learning more about other people, yourself, and life

Caring for a chronically ill person can be a great challenge and opportunity. By entering the sick person's room with an "I don't know what to expect, but I'm here to help in any way I can" attitude, you will be better prepared to meet the person's needs than if you presume to know what to expect (expect the unexpected).

Flexibility, after all, is the name of the game.

45

Honoring Confidences

How very said it is to have a confiding nature;
one's hopes and feelings are quite at the mercy
of all who come along.
—Emily Dickinson

We all need someone to whom we can confide our innermost thoughts and most intimate feelings. This need is especially strong in those who are chronically ill.

A confidence is something said to you in private, for your ears alone, and it should remain private. A confidence is something said that is limited or restricted to the person to whom it is said; it is confidential information and should be protected, never divulged to anyone else.

You must protect confidences—not only because it is the honorable and ethical thing to do, but because to betray a confidence, "even" once, jeopardizes your relationship with the person whose confidence you violated. When you betray a confidence, the person who confided it to you may lose respect for you, becoming unable to trust you from then on.

There are two types of confidences; both should be respected, honored, and safeguarded.

First is the explicit confidence, when someone says to you, "I'm telling this to you in utmost confidence—don't breathe it to a soul."

Second is the implied confidence: the person may not actually say, "hold this in confidence," but the nature of what is said is so obviously of a sensitive and delicate nature that common sense dictates that it must not be repeated to anyone without permission.

Whenever you listen to sensitive information, shared in confidence, it is best to listen in a permissive, nondirective manner; just let the person talk, without probing him or her for details.

After listening to something said in confidence, assure the person that what you have been told will be held in strictest confidence—and be sure that your subsequent behavior matches your pledge.

You may sometimes wish to build a closer relationship by sharing some of your own confidences to build trust. You can encourage the ill individual to feel safe in sharing his or her intimate thoughts and feelings with you if you first reveal some intensely personal things about yourself. In this instance, you give in order to get.

Sometimes you may find it difficult to seal your lips when have strong opinions about something you have been told in confidence, or if you feel that by remaining silent you may endanger the ill person's health or the well-being of other family members. In such situations, think the matter over carefully, considering the consequences of violating, or not violating, the confidence. Consider what is in the best interests of all concerned, and act accordingly. Perhaps the sick person may be contemplating killing himself or herself because of feelings of futility or fear of the future—or perhaps he or she person may be planning to secretly spend a considerable sum of money on something ill-advised, without telling any family members.

The dilemma of whether to honor or divulge a confidence for the good of all concerned must be faced squarely and resolved. But you, and only you, can make this difficult decision. In such a situation, let your conscience be your guide.

46

Paying Attention

Attention is a hard thing to get from men.
—FRANCIS BACON

Effective listening and responding requires that you listen attentively both to what the ill person is actually saying and to what he or she is trying to say. Complete attention—that means 100 percent—is required, because sometimes ill people speak softly or hesitantly, or ramble as they talk. Any of these things can make it difficult to understand what the person is saying.

Try to concentrate completely, focusing yourself totally on what the sick person is saying. You must narrow your perception to a single object—the person who is speaking. Do your best to filter out any competing noise (e.g., television) or distracting activity (e.g., sounds from nearby rooms).

Complete concentration requires your total absorption with what the ill person is saying—it requires that you free your mind of all competing thoughts. Delay your reactions to what is being said, or your thoughts about what you will say in return. This is difficult to do, but it is possible.

You can help yourself in your efforts to listen with complete attention when you

- Keep an open mind
- Are receptive to whatever the person is saying
- Fix your eyes steadily on the face of the person who is speaking
- Place your body so you can see each other easily
- Sit or stand near the person
- Maintain an alert posture
- Shut out any distracting noise
- Remove all physical or visual distractions between you and the ill person

Pay attention to the whole person—to body language, to voice tone and loudness, to choice of words, to rate of speech, to pauses, to silences. When you observe all these things, you will do a better job of hearing what the person is telling you, and you will be able to read between the lines more perceptively.

By giving your full and complete attention to what the ill person is saying, you will improve your chances of understanding what is being said—as the person saying it intended it to be understood.

Partial attention leads to partial hearing, which results in partial understanding. If you are only partially attentive to what an ill person is telling you, your relationship will suffer.

47

Showing Acceptance

I wish they would take me as I am.
—Vincent Van Gogh

Demonstrating your acceptance for someone who is chronically ill is a prerequisite to forming a warm and close relationship with him or her. A seriously ill person craves to be accepted—and, conversely, strongly dislikes being judged by people.

When you accept another person, you take him or her for all that he or she is and is not, without forming any judgments about what he or she says or does. Accepting someone doesn't involve evaluating what her or she says or does as good or bad, right or wrong, or proper or improper.

True acceptance of someone doesn't have anything to do with showing approval or disapproval, or with expressing or implying blame or fault. You simply recognize a person's desirable (and undesirable) qualities and strengths (and weaknesses) without reference to your opinions or judgments about them. By accepting a person, you show your respect for the dignity and worth of that individual. This respect includes acceptance of their thoughts, ideas, feelings, and needs.

Ideally, you will feel unconditional acceptance for an ill person. When you extend unconditional acceptance, you do so without any reservations or qualifications whatso-ever. Granted—this is not an easy thing to do.

When a seriously ill person feels accepted, he or she feels safe, liked, even prized. He or she feels free to experi-ence himself or herself as a person who has all kinds of thoughts and feelings, and has no need to feel defensive or guilty about them. Your acceptance of a person allows him or her to honestly discuss whatever he or she wishes, whenever and however he or she desires.

When someone who is sick finds someone who accepts his or her thoughts and feelings without feeling the need to judge them, he or she is better able to listen to himself or herself, and to become more self-aware. For example, someone who is sick may become able to admit that he or she is depressed, angry, or frightened, and may feel less inclined to deny or repress such thoughts and feelings. Actively encouraging someone who is ill to express his or her innermost thoughts and feelings to you is extremely helpful—and when this happens, it is essential that you acknowledge that you have heard what the person has said.

You can show a person that you accept him or her by
- Being there when he or she needs you most
- Touching him or her
- Standing or sitting close to hand

- Acting comfortable and relaxed when you're around him or her
- Being thoughtful, and helping him or her as much as you can
- Being supportive, reassuring, and empowering
- Expressing your liking for him or her, and the pleasure you derive from spending time together
- Showing him or her that what he or she says and does is important to you
- Refraining from trying to change his or her beliefs and ways of doing things
- Listening carefully and lovingly to what he or she says
- Showing that you respect and admire him or her as a person
- Exuding patience and concern during trying situations
- Talking about, and listening him or her talk about, things he or she is interested in
- Sharing his or her pain and sorrow
- Laughing and kidding around together

It is not enough merely to accept a person as he or she is as well as for what he or she is becoming—you must be sure to demonstrate your acceptance clearly. Someone who is ill needs to know that you accept him or her. Your total being (your voice, your choice of words, your body language, and everything else about you) must all be consistent in thundering your acceptance of such a person.

But make no mistake: perhaps the greatest challenge you will face when accepting an ill person is permitting the person to be hostile toward you, allowing him or her to vent anger on you. Doing this requires considerable self-control. Becoming an accepting person is hard work, but you will find it easier to accept others once you have been able to accept yourself. Your acceptance of others begins with self-acceptance.

48

Showing Empathy

Two souls with but a single thought,
two hearts that beat as one.
—Maria Lovell

Possessing and demonstrating compassion and empathy is essential to forming a warm, close relationship with someone who is ill.

There are two aspects of empathy:

1. Accurately sensing an ill person's thoughts and feelings.
2. Conveying this understanding to the ill person.

You have empathy when you perceive the world in a way similar to that in which an ill person sees it, seeing the sick individual much as he or she views himself or herself. In doing so, you are able to achieve an internal frame of reference similar to that of the ailing person.

An empathetic person accepts the fact that people basically have to act as they do—whether it be good, or bad.

Try your best to see things from the other person's point of view, but recognize that no one is able to fully understand another person; each of us is unique, with different life experiences and a different way of perceiving things. But you do have the potential to visualize yourself in the ill person's situation. Ask yourself, "How might I think, feel, or behave in similar circumstances?" or "What might I be tempted to say or do if I were in the other person's situation?"

Conveying empathy for a person helps the ill person feel safe and understood because he or she finds that whatever attitude, thoughts, or feelings he or she expresses are understood almost exactly as he or she perceives them.

You feel compassion for someone when you are conscious of his or her difficulties, and when you desire to alleviate the stress he or she is experiencing. You have a warm feeling for the person, and exhibit feelings of tenderness and sympathy for his or her plight. You demonstrate compassion for a person when you

- Strive to promote the person's dignity and value as a person
- Make the person feel important and needed, making him or her feel like a somebody
- Help the person keep control of his or her own life (for example, by allowing him or her to make decisions)
- Keep him or her involved in daily life as appropriate (for example, in family activities)

- Are aware of the person's right—and need—to know important things, and when you accept your responsibility to provide such information
- Level with the person when providing information—without leveling the person in the process
- Are objective when dealing with the facts, but are also compassionate in dealing with the person
- Calmly and graciously accept criticism, even angry outbursts, from the person
- Let the person vent and blow off steam to you
- Take care to say the special, endearing things you want to say when they should be said, rather than waiting until it is too late
- Refrain from saying certain things whose consequences would be grave and serve no useful purpose

You perform an outstanding service to those who are ill when you show them you have empathy and compassion for them and their problems.

49

Showing Respect

*He removes the greatest ornament of friendship
who takes away from it respect.*
—Cicero

Respect and trust form the basis of any enduring,
meaningful relationship. It is axiomatic that without
respect you can't have a worthwhile relationship.

When you respect a person, you

- Hold him or her in high regard
- Admire and have great esteem for him or her
- Honor and look up to him or her
- Appreciate and value him or her
- Treat him or her as a person first, and as someone
  who is sick second

You can demonstrate your respect for a seriously ill
person in a number of ways. Make it clear that you consider him or her important, and that his or her life still has
purpose and is worth living despite the illness.

Show that you consider him or her competent to still
do many things on his or her own; do this by asking for his

or her ideas, advice, and suggestions on various matters. And when he or she obliges, consider what he or she says carefully, and then follow up on whatever is practical. Ask and listen to his or her opinions about family matters and world events. Include him or her in family decision-making and activities. And—which is crucial—help him or her feel that he or she is still in control of his or her own life, and responsible for it.

Convey your respect by putting your sick friend or loved one first. Make yourself available when you are needed instead of only when it is convenient for you to help. Listen more than you talk. Pay total attention when you listen, and then respond appropriately to what has been said. Hear the person out rather than interrupting, cutting off discussion, or changing the subject when you want to. Also, listen patiently—refrain from rushing conversations.

In addition, show your respect by cooperating with the individual as much as possible. Be willing to go the extra mile for him or her. Try to give him or her choices, and accede to his or her wishes whenever feasible. Do things the way he or she wants them done as much as is practical; for example, don't change the room's furnishings or daily routines without prior discussion, and without winning agreement on the changes. Also, be courteous; request permission before entering his or her room. This will show you respect his or her privacy.

Seek opportunities to build the person's confidence and feelings of self-worth. Let him or her know that you feel honored to be around him or her, and grateful for the opportunity to help out. Give praise freely whenever warranted. Don't criticize unless it is absolutely necessary. And when criticism is necessary, do it in the least objectionable manner.

Help the person by being positive rather than negative. Avoid any put-downs. Don't express sarcasm or engage in ridicule. And when you need to disagree, show respect by doing it politely and tactfully.

Try to get on the same wavelength and talk *with* the person—not *at* the person. Speak as equals, and from a viewpoint that says that you are both okay. Provide an opportunity for the person to state his or her wishes and preferences on matters that are important to him or her. Make a sincere effort to understand his or her wishes by getting feedback, and by reading between the lines if necessary.

Learn what is important to him or her—the things he or she likes and dislikes. For example, use his or her preferred name, and take his or her complaints and criticisms seriously, following up on them as appropriate. If you need to request that he or she do something, make sure that he or she perceives it as a request, and not as a demand.

By keeping an ill person fully (and promptly) informed, you can demonstrate respect for him or her. It is especially important that you give him or her advanced notice of anything that will significantly affect his or her life. When providing such notice, do it sincerely and truthfully. You are obligated to share all relevant information—uncensored. Show your respect by talking candidly.

Provide privacy whenever you need to discuss anything personal or sensitive in nature. Show your respect by keeping everything said in confidence to you strictly confidential.

As is true of everyone, someone who is ill needs to get rid of pent-up emotions from time to time. Convey your respect by encouraging the person to frankly utter what things on his or her mind are causing him or her to feel frustrated. And when he or she unleashes his or her emotions, pay close attention, and be willing to act as a sponge or punching bag. Respect his or her right to be upset. While listening, stay calm, and don't take anything personally. And finally, show your respect by doing meaningful things together.

50

Showing Understanding

Each of us needs to understand himself and
understand others and be taken care of himself.
—HANIEL LONG

Seek not only to be understood, but to understand. Most of us tend to concentrate on getting ourselves understood by others, yet it is just as important to understand others. It is hard work and requires expending considerable energy to understand someone else—especially since it is impossible to ever wholly and completely understand exactly what another person has said to us. However, you can understand an ill person best if you attempt to view things from his or her perspective and try to see things as he or she sees them.

Every ill person has something worthwhile to say and should be listened to. However, gravely ill people may not be able to think of words to accurately describe what they are experiencing and trying to tell you. In such instances, be willing to make every effort to understand what an ill person is trying to say to you.

Making accurate interpretations of something said to you is especially difficult when the ill person is disoriented and speaking in a rambling manner. Also, it is easy to misunderstand what an ill person is trying to say to you, because his or her utterance may often be obscure, only partially stated, or expressed in symbolic language (e.g., dreams or stories about past events).

You must have realistic expectations when talking with any seriously ill person; even well people seldom say exactly what is on their mind. Regrettably, you can't ever realistically expect to completely understand another person, because no two people see and hear things the same way. We are all unique beings with different perceptions, and with different ways of saying and interpreting things. What is obvious to you may be totally obscure and unclear to someone else, and vice versa.

Even slight variation in the words expressed can cause minor to major differences in how the words are interpreted and reacted to. The difficulty in gaining understanding is compounded by the need to understand not only the meaning of an ill person's words, but the feelings behind their use.

But you can't afford to dismiss the ramblings of an ill person just because they make little or no sense to you. Nor can you talk down to him or her and treat him or her as a child; this strips him or her of dignity and creates resentment. Treating an ill person appropriately requires awareness, desire, and persistence to make sense of some of the things he or she says to you. To decipher what an ill person is saying, pay attention not only to the words he or she uses, but to his or her facial expressions, tone of voice, and gestures.

What appears to be confused, aimless talk can be significant. By decoding these apparently obscure messages, you can relieve some of the ill person's distress and anxiety. Why? Because he or she is likely desperate to be understood.

It is vital that you not only understand an ill person, but also *show* him or her you understand him or her. He or she needs to know, to have reassurance, that you understand him or her. You can show that you understand what a person has said to you by the things you say, and the things you do, in response. If an ill person tells you about severe pain or states that he or she is feeling very sad and you fail to react appropriately, with a concerned look on your face or an empathetic comment, the person could interpret this as in undesirable ways:

- "You must not have gotten my message."
- "You don't care about me or my feelings."

Your understanding of other people will be enhanced by your self-understanding. Each of us has his or her own emotional blind spots, prejudices, and hang-ups, concerns, fears, and preferences, all of which differ from those of others. We must become aware of these. There are several specific, tangible ways that you can show that you understand an ill person's comments and feelings:

- Restate in your own words what the person has said. Simply rephrase the key thoughts or feelings stated by the sick individual: "As I understand it, you are really feeling down today because you are feeling a sense of futility about your condition." It is important to note that merely mirroring back (using the same words) what a person has said to you does not show that you understand, but only that you are able to repeat the words spoken to you.

- Ask probing questions related to what you've been told to clarify or seek more information on some point: "Would you tell me more about why you feel that your condition is hopeless?"

- Make the following kinds of statements (doing so doesn't guarantee that you truly understand what was said, but is reassuring to a chronically ill person): "I see," "I hear you," "I understand," "I share your concern."

- Make reassuring sounds without saying any words: "Hmm."

- Exhibit facial expressions that are compatible with what the person is saying to you, in conjunction with an appropriate body position: a frown, a sad look, a nod, a steady look and concerned expression.

- Cite a related anecdote or story.

- Informally summarize key points at the end of the discussion: "Let me see if I have this right—the main reasons you feel your condition is improving are . . ."

- Follow up appropriately on what was said, or fulfill a request made of you.

Your relationship with an ill person will greatly improve when you understand, and demonstrate that you understand, his or her needs, wants, concerns, interests, anxieties, fears, and thoughts on important matters.

51

Sizing Up Moods

Things are not always as they seem.
—Phaedrus

The more quickly and accurately you are able to size up an ill person, the better. It is important to size up a person correctly so that you will know how best to deal with him or her. However, try to avoid being obvious when doing so, because people resent being evaluated.

When you size up someone, you form an opinion, or make judgments, about him or her. You try to figure out what makes the person tick; you try to take their measure. You attempt to ascertain the person's attitudes, character, beliefs, and ability. In addition, you try to determine what things are important, and unimportant, to him or her.

By sizing up certain things, you will be able to relate to, and understand, a seriously ill person better:

- Personality traits—for example, introvert/extrovert, trusting/suspicious, optimistic/pessimistic, confident/insecure
- Strength of convictions—for example, flexible/rigid
- Prejudices and pet peeves

- Mood indicators—facial expressions, body language, voice clues
- Extent of knowledge and general understanding of things
- Attitude toward illness—for example, acceptance/ rejection, desire to be independent/willingness to be helped
- General intelligence and ability to comprehend events
- Receptivity to change—for example, open-/closed-mindedness.
- Thinking style: for example, fast/slow
- Morning/evening person
- Energy/fatigue
- Talker/listener
- Important spiritual values (or lack thereof)
- Attitude toward people generally, and you specifically

Now that you are familiar with several of the important things to size up, let's explore various ways you can go about sizing up a chronically ill person:

- Free up your own mind, and open up all your senses.
- Observe all aspects of the person's behavior—for example, the things he or she does, and how and when he or she does them.
- Remain silent and listen carefully. Talk only to ask relevant questions.
- Note the person's appearance—is he or she unkempt, or well groomed?

- Notice the person's vocabulary level and choice of words.
- Observe the person's voice characteristics—for example, strong/weak, loud/quiet, lively/dull, expressive/monotone.
- Be aware of the person's body position—for example, relaxed/tense.
- Watch the person's body movements and gestures—for example, frequent and free/infrequent and up tight.
- Notice facial expressions—for example, animated/frozen, spontaneous/contrived, expressive/guarded.
- Read between the lines for contradictions between words and facial expressions or body movement.
- Notice the extent the person is self-centered versus other-centered by observing the frequency in which he or she says *I*, *me*, and *my*, compared with *you*, in his or her conversation.
- Pay attention to the topics he or she introduces in conversation—for example, does he or she talk primarily about his or her physical condition? his or her family? the community? the nation? Learn how big his or her world is.
- Observe what he or she does and doesn't react to—and how strongly.
- Notice any significant changes in what he or she says or does.
- Ask for the opinions of others who know him or her well.

It is important not only to size up a person overall, but to size him or her up at particular times so that you can assess his or her mood at a particular moment. By knowing his or her mood, you can adapt what you say and do to it.

To assess a person's mood, notice

- How he or she greets you—warmly, or with disinterest
- Anything different or noteworthy about his or her appearance
- His or her body position—for example, standing, sitting, or lying down
- His or her reactions to your initial comments or questions
- His or her facial expressions
- The extent of energy he or she displays—for example, lively/lethargic
- The nature of his or her comments or questions
- The volume, pitch, and variation of his or her voice
- His or her reaction to your visit—receptive, or preoccupied

To relate and communicate most effectively with an ill person, you need to know who he or she really is rather than simply who he or she appears to be. And you need to know his or her mood at particular times. You can gain these important insights by sizing him or her up accurately. The results are well worth the effort.

PART 5

RESPONDING

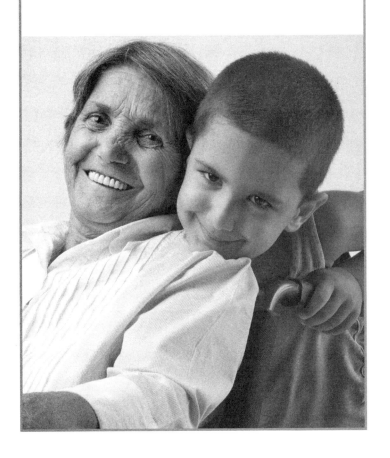

52

Responding to Anger

There never was an angry man that thought his anger unjust.
—Saint Francis de Sales

Anger is a natural, normal human emotion. We all become angry on occasion. A chronically ill person may, understandably, be short-tempered more frequently than a well person—especially if he or she is feeling uncomfortable or is in pain. People are also more likely to behave aggressively when they are feeling discouraged, frustrated, or frightened—emotions all too common in those who are seriously ill.

Anger can be either creative or destructive. Expressing anger can be a positive force for change, because it can energize a person enough to deal with his or her frustrations and problems. But suppressed anger can cause problems in relationships, and can cause depression. Pent-up anger is like poison in a person's system, and like poison, it can interfere with the healing process.

Once anger is expressed and acknowledged, it dissipates—and anger must be allowed to subside before any meaningful discussion of the feelings associated with the anger can occur. In addition to discussing a person's feelings and their causes, it is sometimes helpful for the person who was recently angry to write down some of the feeling he or she experienced when angry. Simply identifying these feelings, and their causes, can be therapeutic.

When a person experiences feelings of anger, he or she often directs the anger at other people, or at things. In some instances, you may well be the target of such anger.

Someone who is angry can behave in insulting and abusive ways. And when someone is attacked by someone who is angry, he or she typically feels stressed. His or her blood pressure increases, and his or her body secretes adrenalin. When you are attacked, you will instinctively want either to fight back or to flee, perhaps both physically and psychologically. If you give into an impulse to fight, you may say something in the heat of the moment that you will later regret. But if you simply give in to an impulse to fight, you may suppress your feelings, say nothing at all, or even turn and walk away.

Although you can't control an ill person's anger, you can control the way you respond to it. You must stay calm and self-controlled; don't get excited or respond in angry. Monitor your feelings, remembering the three Cs: be calm, be cool, be collected. Refuse to let someone who is angry person push your buttons. You and you alone are responsible for controlling your own emotions. Before acting in the heat of the moment, pause a second to consider the consequences of what you are considering saying or doing.

After the angry episode is over, consider how the situation could be avoided in the future. Do your best to put yourself in the other person's position. Ask yourself, "As he or she perceived it, was there a legitimate reason for the anger?" And since anger is merely a symptom, look for the cause of the anger, realizing that a person's long-term illness involves many unknowns as well as considerable uncertainty—both of which create anxiety and fear within a person.

Anger doesn't occur in a vacuum. It is triggered by other emotions and perceptions, such as feelings of helplessness, resentment, and rejection. Try to discover whether there are any recurring incidents that trigger the angry outbursts. By identifying these causes, you can better predict the times and situations when the person might get angry—and then try to avoid them. For example, do certain persons or events seem to provoke the anger? If so, take appropriate preventative action.

If you learn that the cause of the anger is a feeling of helplessness, deal with those feelings directly rather than with the anger, which is only a symptom. You might say, "Having to ask for help so much right now is really frustrating to you, isn't it?"

But let the person feel anger, and let him or her show it. Let him or her vent—this is his or her right. The expression of anger is therapeutic, and will help him or her feel better.

But never ignore or dismiss an ill person's anger, and don't try to downplay it. If someone who is ill asks, "What have I done to deserve this? Why has God done this to me?" it would be a grave mistake to reply, "That's a lot of nonsense—you know God isn't doing this to you!"

Make yourself strong enough to allow an angry person to attack you verbally and take out his or her frustrations on you. Although he or she may be upset with someone or something else entirely, you may be the only available target.

If the person's anger really is directed elsewhere, don't take the attack personally or take offense. Instead, listen attentively and patiently, with understanding. And if the anger directed toward you is justified, admit that you acted improperly. Assume responsibility, and take the appropriate action to resolve the problem, apologizing sincerely and making the necessary changes to remedy the situation.

Here is a good method for dealing with someone who is angry:

- Listen in a friendly, interested manner.
- Make your sincere concern evident.
- Stay calm, maintaining your self-control (never argue or say or do anything in retaliation).
- Acknowledge the person's feelings, and assure him or her of your concern because of his or her anger. You might say, "I can see you're really angry about this. I'll listen—why don't you tell me all about it?"
- Listen with total concentration, and with an open

mind. Pay attention to his or her feelings, as well as to the facts and words expressed.

- Hear the person out—let him or her say everything he or she wants to say without interrupting. (If you try to interrupt or to defend yourself while someone is still angry, you will likely just make matters worse.)

- Wait for the person to finish saying what he or she has to say before you attempt to say anything substantial yourself. (You can tell when the time is right by waiting until the person's body relaxes and his or her voice changes.)

- Make reflective (mirroring) comments about the feelings the person expresses to show you have heard him or her. Echo in your own words the feelings and facts he or she has expressed regarding the causes of his or her anger. For example, you might say, "I can understand your feeling upset because your best friend did not visit you like she promised," or "Oh, I understand why you're so upset—is it because . . ."

- Ask a few brief questions after the person is through venting in order to clarify your own understanding, or to learn more about something he or she said.

- Respond calmly and in a conversational tone of voice (remember—"a soft answer turneth away wrath"). Refrain from making any judgmental statements, as well as from acting defensive or coming on too strong. Instead, say something like, "I don't blame you for being upset—your friends' visits are very important to you."

- Try to propose a solution that is satisfactory to the angry person: "Would you like for me to invite your friend to have lunch with you tomorrow?"
- Look for the causes of the anger rather than focusing on the anger alone. For example, did the ill person feel rejected because he or she was excluded from a family party?
- If the anger is excessive and you feel as though you are close to losing your self-control, don't hesitate to leave the room. Simply say, "I'm sorry—I need to leave now, but I'll come back in a bit."

Remember—the words you speak are like bullets: once fired, they can't be recalled, and they can cause deep and permanent wounds. And although people may forgive a hurt, they may never be able to forget it.

53

Responding to Complaints

Complain to one who can help you.
—Yugoslav Proverb

It is natural for chronically ill people to have complaints from time to time. This is to be expected. All complaints need to be dealt with conscientiously, whether they are legitimate or not.

It is important to recognize that imagined complaints are just as serious to a sick person as are real ones. Such complaints can be very real to an ill person.

There are generally two things on the mind of the complaining party:

1. What is wrong
2. What you are going to do about it

Conversely, a person listening to a complaint typically has three concerns:

1. What, generally, is wrong
2. What, specifically, is wrong
3. How the matter can be resolved to the satisfaction of the person who is complaining

The following attitudes and practices have proven successful when dealing with complaints:

- Listen in a friendly manner, rather than being uptight and defensive.
- Try to provide privacy while the complaint is aired.
- Hear the person out—don't rush him or her.
- Listen attentively, and with an open mind.
- Refrain from interrupting the person—let him or her get rid of all the anger in his or her system before you say anything.
- After the person has calmed down, ask him or her to clarify anything that is unclear to you—for example, "Would you tell me more about why you feel neglected?"
- By repeating the complaint, acknowledge that you understand it—for example, "As I understand it, you feel neglected and strongly resent it."
- Pay special attention to the feelings expressed, and to how intensely they are felt. Don't make the mistake of listening only to the facts stated.
- Express your concern for the discomfort, associated with the complaint, that the person is experiencing.
- Set limits on how much you talk when responding. Perceptive listening, not lengthy response, is the key to handling complaints successfully.

After showing the person that you understand the complaint and demonstrating your sincere concern, you can do one of three things:

1. If the complaint is legitimate, grant that it is warranted, and state what you can do to rectify the matter. Also, pledge that you will do your best to see that the problem is not repeated.

2. If you need to think about the complaint or secure more information before responding, say something like: "I understand the problem, but I need to look into the matter more fully before I can do anything. Let me get back to you tomorrow." It is essential that you state the time the person can expect an answer so he or she won't feel left hanging. Be sure to give an answer by the promised time.

3. If the complaint clearly is unfounded or is based on incorrect information, diplomatically explain the facts and the actual situation so that you can put the matter in the true perspective for the complaining person.

Use a calm, conversational tone of voice when explaining the facts. Refrain from acting in an aggressive or abrupt manner, and never just dismiss the complaint as being of no merit. Instead, it is a good idea to emphasize the facts related to the complaint, deemphasizing who was right and who was wrong.

It is important to protect the ill person's self-esteem by avoiding the use of the words "you were wrong." Instead, say something like: "If I had the same understanding of the facts as you did, I'd probably be angry too. But let me explain things as I believe they really are."

It is imperative that you realize that sometimes when ill people are complaining about something, they are not really seeking a solution to their complaint. Rather, they are seeking to be noticed, to be listened to, and to get pent-up frustrations aired and off their chest. You, in turn, must be sensitive and perceptive enough to detect the real motivation behind an ill person's complaint.

54

Responding to Crying

Sir, there is no crying for shed milk.
That which is past cannot be recalled.
—ANDREW YARRANTON

It is okay to cry. Crying is normal and common—a thing people do. Sometimes ill people need to cry. Crying is a good thing, because it is both healing and therapeutic; it can be as beneficial as laughter. Since crying provides emotional release, it should be encouraged, not discouraged.

Permit an ill person to cry—give him or her full license to do so. Say, and show, that it is okay for a person to cry. And note that even men should feel free to cry. Neither men nor women need to feel ashamed or embarrassed when crying.

It is important to realize that crying is not an emotion—it is a symptom. Depending on the situation, crying can be a symptom of various emotions such as fright, anger, frustration, sadness, despair, depression, and pain, among countless others.

Crying is not weakness! Neither the person who is crying or a person who is witnessing the crying should feel bothered by it. People who never cry are emotionally deficient and incomplete. Thus, it is unwise and uncaring to stifle the crying of a person who needs to cry.

Most of us are not good at coping with others' tears. We feel uncomfortable, and we don't know how to react. We may want to do something comforting, but we don't know what to do, or how to do it.

The most comforting thing you can do for someone who is crying is simply to be present, and to listen when the person is ready to speak. Don't feel compelled to say or do anything while the person is sobbing. It is best to observe calmly, quietly, and compassionately, without acting uncomfortable. Let the person get all cried out without interfering with the emotional release. Usually the person will stop crying on his or her own when he or she no longer feels the need to cry, so you don't need to do anything to help him or her to stop. However, in rare instances of prolonged, uncontrolled crying, you may need to seek the help of some kind of health professional; this is a serious matter.

Be careful how you react to crying, and be sure to respond appropriately. Here are several ideas that you may find helpful when reacting to a person's crying:

- Be flexible, and ready to adapt what you say or do to the individual involved and the particular situation.

- Realize that you didn't cause the person to cry (if this is indeed the case), so there is no need for you to act anxious or defensive.
- Refrain from saying anything supportive that may interrupt the person's crying—let him or her finish crying before you say or do anything (except perhaps provide a tissue if needed).
- Recognize that the person needs to pour out his or her grief before he or she can move on.
- Be willing to share his or her sadness by empathizing.
- Feel free to show some emotion yourself, including a few tears—you are a compassionate human being, not an unresponsive machine.
- Give the crying process plenty of time—don't do anything to rush it.
- Be careful not to say anything to negate or minimize the person's feelings. It would be presumptuous for you to tell the person what he or she should and shouldn't feel—for example, by saying, "Come now, that's nothing for you to feel bad about."
- Sit silently and attentively while the person is crying.
- Don't feel obligated to make any suggestions or offer any solutions related to the crying—your presence is the crucial thing.
- After the person is finished crying, ask him or her if he or she wants to be alone, to be with you only, or to be with several other people to discuss his or her reasons for crying.

- Offer to help in any way you can, whether now or later.
- Make a brief, helpful comment or two later in the conversation, if appropriate.

As emphasized earlier, the best way to comfort a crying person depends on the particular person, on your relationship with the person, and on the circumstances involved. But the following sequence of steps is recommended for most people in most circumstances:

1. Move close to the person and sit side by side.
2. Show the person by your actions that it is okay to cry, and that you are there for him or her.
3. Offer a tissue quickly and without comment, if needed.
4. Listen patiently until the person is through crying.
5. Touch the person reassuringly to comfort him or her without impeding the flow of tears.
6. Encourage the person, without being insistent, to tell about the emotion causing the crying—if he or she wants to.
7. Make supportive and compassionate comments at appropriate times.
8. Stay with the person until he or she gets calm and regains his or her composure—unless he or she expresses a desire to be alone.
9. Ask for specific ways you can help before you leave.

A couple of topics deserve further mention—touching and talking. Touching is desirable to show caring and support, but it should be done in such a way that doesn't indicate that it is time for the crying to stop. Touching is helpful, because it is soothing and reassuring. A quick hug or timely holding of hands is reassuring, but it should not impede the person's crying.

It is important for you to talk at the right time. All your comments should be delayed until the person has finished crying and shows that he or she is ready to talk. You will need to sense when the person is ready to talk. It is all right to ask questions in a low-key fashion to try to identify the reasons for crying, if and when you consider it appropriate to do so. But be careful not to pressure the person to talk until he or she is fully ready to do so. It is sometimes helpful to discuss something comparable that happened to you in order to create a greater spirit of understanding and togetherness.

Let the other person do most of the talking and lead the discussion (e.g., choose the topics to discuss) before entering into the give-and-take phase of the conversation.

Certain statements you can make to a crying person are helpful, and others are harmful. It is important both that you say the right things and that you avoid saying the wrong things:

Helpful Statements

- "I hear what you're saying."
- "I understand."
- "Go ahead and cry—let it all out."
- "Remember, I'm here for you."
- " I can see you're really hurting."
- "You must be feeling terrible."
- "You're not alone in this."

Harmful Statements

- "Things can't be that bad."
- "Stop being a baby."
- "You need to be brave."
- "Come now—compose yourself."
- "Crying isn't going to help anything."
- "I can't understand why you are crying about something like that."
- "There's no point in crying—you can't do anything about it."
- "Don't you think you're making a mountain out of a molehill?"

We all need to cry at one time or another. This is a part of the human condition. Crying is honorable, healthful, and nothing to be ashamed about. We need to feel free to cry when we need to, and to feel comfortable while doing it. And we need to become more comfortable when we are around others who are crying.

Remember: truly strong people are able to cry.

55

Responding to Depression

Those who are unhappy have no need for anything in the
world but people capable of giving them their attention.
—Simone Weil

Feeling depressed on occasion is a normal part of being
seriously ill; feelings of sadness and futility are to be
expected at times. However, any feelings and expressions
of depression should be acknowledged, accepted, and
respected. These feelings should never be joked about or
dismissed, because to do so would be insulting, and would
show a lack of compassion for the person.

Symptoms of depression commonly include:

- Irritation
- Loss of interest or pleasure in most activities
- Significant weight loss/gain or appetite increase/
  decrease
- Insomnia
- Declining ability to think and concentrate
- Recurrent and excessive negative thoughts

A depressed person typically expresses one or more of the following emotions:

- loneliness
- lostness
- rejection
- discouragement
- hopelessness
- disappointment
- sadness
- feeling "down"
- hurt
- feeling crushed
- emptiness
- vulnerability
- feeling used
- confusion
- boredom
- feeling abused
- isolation
- feeling wronged

You will need to let the depressed person express his or her feelings without making any judgments about them. It's a mistake to try to pressure a depressed person to explain why he or she feels the way he or she does; simply accept the fact that he or she feels depressed.

There can be many reasons why an ill person may be depressed. Depression is often caused by feelings of futility and grief, for example, over what the person has already lost due to his or her illness, or what he or she may lose in the future. The person may feel sad because he or she feels trapped. Such a person may often feel overwhelmed by his or her predicament, and by the fact that he or she has lost the ability to control his or her life. Another common cause of sadness is the feeling that he or she has become a burden to his or her friends and loved ones.

Regrettably, there is not much you can do to relieve an ill person's feelings of depression. Your attempts to cheer up or reassure the person mean very little, and your words usually have minimum affect. The person is hard to reach, because he or she is hurting deep inside. His or her biggest need is to express his or her sorrow freely and fully, without any hindrance. Someone who is depressed feels best when he or she perceives that he or she is being listened to by an empathetic person.

So what can you do to help? First of all, just listen. Simply listen, and keep listening as long as the person wants to talk. Listen to the person's pain. Share the feelings of pain by looking concerned. Show your compassion by your body language and facial expressions. Touch the person in the right way, at the right time. Be careful to avoid looking judgmentally or saying anything judgmental.

The best thing is to truly listen, to let the person express his or her sadness fully. After hearing the person out, you can reflect, or mirror, the person's expressed feelings. For example, "You are really feeling sad about things today." Be sure to say this with a caring look and in a compassionate tone of voice. You could also ask sincerely, "Is there anything I can do to help you feel better?" But perhaps the most powerful thing you can do is to touch the person in a loving, reassuring manner.

The most important thing for you to convey to a depressed person about his or her sadness is, *I'm here for you, no matter what happens.*

Much as you would like to help the depressed person feel better, you don't need to feel responsible for making him or her feel better, nor obligated to relieve his or her grief. The remedy is out of your hands, and beyond your ability to control.

However, there are some things you should avoid saying to a depressed person, because by saying them you could make things worse. Beware of saying anything trite or flippant, or that makes light of the person's feelings:

- "You shouldn't talk like that."
- "Try to look on the bright side of things."
- "You'll feel better tomorrow."
- "Cheer up! Things could be a lot worse."
- "Come now—things can't be all *that* bad."
- "Be thankful you've had such a long and happy life."
- "It hurts me to hear you say things like that."

It is also ill-advised to act impatient or irritated by the sad things you're being told. Additionally, it is a mistake to interrupt the person, or to change the subject, and it is nothing less than heartless to joke around about the person's mood.

It can't be emphasized too much—the best thing you can do is to listen, to listen again, and then to listen some more.

56

Responding to Personal Attacks and Insults

It is often better not to see an insult than to avenge it.
—Seneca

Regrettably, you must expect, on occasion, to suffer verbal attacks and insults from an ailing individual.

It is important for you to try to understand the reasons for these hostile actions. The reasons may include the following:

- You have done something the ill person considers offensive.
- The person is in a bad mood, and is irritable.
- The person is in pain, and instinctively lashes out at the only person present.
- The person may be adversely affected by his or her medicines, and unable to control his or her emotions.
- The person feels constant anger and resentment over his or her illness.

There are a number of acceptable responses to an ill person's attacks on you, but there is also a completely unacceptable response—losing your cool and retaliating with equally insulting remarks or hostile actions.

The acceptable responses range from a soft, loving response to immediate departure from the room. You must select the most appropriate response for the particular situation. Possible responses include

- Ignoring the attack and doing nothing—just listening to the person vent
- Touching the person in a loving way—turning the other cheek (e.g., you could say, "You can say whatever you want to, but I still like you.")
- Acknowledging the insult, and responding kindly to the feelings expressed
- Checking out the cause—if you discover you have done something offensive, apologize and express your regret
- Making a neutral statement such as, "I'm sorry you feel that way"; this kind of statement expresses regret without accepting any blame
- Leaving the room, and as you are leaving, saying, "I'll be back later" (do this only if the insults are extremely abusive and the anger excessive; later, after the person has calmed down, if the attack was directed at you personally, quietly defend yourself and state the reasons you felt the insults were unwarranted); if the insults are persistent over a period of

time, you may need to set boundaries for acceptable and unacceptable behavior and discuss these with the ill person so that they are clearly understood

None of us likes to be the brunt of insulting, abusive behavior, but some venting of hostility by chronically ill people is to be expected. Because of this, we need to practice self-control, to learn how to best deal with this offensive behavior whenever it is exhibited.

57

Responding to Repetitive Statements

True humanity consists not in a squeamish ear;
it consists not in starting or shrinking at tales of misery,
but in a disposition of heart to relieve it.
—Charles Fox

Many chronically ill people become forgetful and sometimes say the same thing over and over again. Typically they do not realize that they keep repeating themselves. You need to know how to deal with these situations. Listening to the same statement and answering questions time and again can become both annoying and downright frustrating. You will be required to show considerable patience and understanding.

Try to identify the reasons for the repetitive statements or questions. You need to understand the cause of the problem before you can deal with it effectively. There are many possibilities:

- It may be a symptom of the illness itself.
- The topic may be of particular importance to the person.

- Something may be on the person's mind that needs to be resolved.
- The person may feel that you haven't heard or responded to a concern he or she has expressed.
- The person may simply be seeking reassurance about the matter.

There are several ways you can respond to a person's repetitive statements and questions. The approach you use depends, naturally, on the cause of the problem.

Here are several responses you may want to consider:

- Listen politely but without saying anything.
- Tactfully try to change the subject.
- Give brief, polite acknowledgements or answers.
- Smile and touching the person's arm while nodding and making a *hmm* sound.
- Ask succinct questions each time, showing that you understand it.
- Say, "I understand," in a kindly manner.
- Say, "We've talked about this several times now; is there something I'm missing that you'd like to tell me more about?"
- Say, "I know this is very important to you—what's going on?" For example: "Mom, I know you've been wondering where your cat is right now—what are you feeling when you think about it?"

It is a bad idea to merely ignore and dismiss repetitive comments or questions. Such a reaction is unkind, and lacks compassion. Nor is it helpful to simply say, "You just told me that"—the person may not remember what he or she has just finished saying. In trying situations such as these, patience is what is needed.

58

Responding to Spiritual Concerns

I can do all things through Christ which strengthens me.
—Philippians 4:13

Some degree of spiritual anxiety is natural to someone who is seriously ill. Being ill creates great uncertainty, and with it fear of the unknown. A seriously ill person is often eager to come to terms with his or her own mortality; he or she may need to fill a vacuum in his or her life that can only be filled by spirituality. In such times, such a person may have many perplexing questions he or she needs addressed.

It is hard for people to talk about spirituality per se; this is because it is intangible, and can't be entirely reduced to rational concepts that can be fully expressed or completely understood. Regrettably, some spiritual questions do not have simple, easy answers—even when asked of an experienced theologian.

It is important to realize that spiritual needs are not the same as religious needs. Spiritual needs are universal in nature, and address issues such as nurturing and the sources of personal solace. The spiritual aspects of a serious illness concern a person's search for the meaning of his or her illness, the meaning of his or her life, and his or her future, including after death. An ill person's suffering can be unbearable without a fundamental understanding of these vital issues. The all-consuming question for a seriously ill person is: what else is there? A common fear is that of not existing, or of no longer being.

Discussing spirituality with an ill person can be difficult, because it requires that you first understand the sick person's needs before you can offer any spiritual help. This challenge is compounded by the fact that spiritual distress is sometimes hard to distinguish from psychological or emotional distress.

Because it can be easy to miss or ignore spiritual pain, be alert to its signs. Note, too, that sometimes relieving a person's spiritual pain requires alleviating his or her physical pain as well.

It is essential that you understand your role in discussing spiritual matters; some spirituality topics are so complex that most lay persons should not attempt to deal with them. If you attempt to help with these complex issues when you don't have the knowledge or skills required to do so helpfully, you could do more harm than good, increasing the person's confusion even as you deprive him or her of desperately needed help from a knowledgeable theologian.

If your spiritual knowledge is inadequate to meet the needs of the person for whom you are caring, don't be afraid to recognize, and openly admit, that certain spiritual needs and questions are beyond your ability to discuss meaningfully and answer intelligently. In such an instance, you can form a partnership with a minister, a priest, or a rabbi who can provide truly effective spiritual help to the seriously ill person for whom you are caring. Don't feel that you yourself must possess all spiritual knowledge required to help the person for whom you are caring; don't hesitate to call for help when it is needed. If you don't have the knowledge necessary to help spiritually, don't try to merely wing it—you can do too much harm if you don't know what you're doing.

But no matter what your spiritual training is, you have an appropriate role to play when it comes to spiritual matters:

- Be a confidant and a source of support.
- Listen attentively, rather than shutting the person down with a harsh, judgmental attitude.
- Ask clarifying questions in response to comments made to you; for example, "Would you tell me what you meant when you said . . ."
- Provide an opportunity for the person to speak freely.
- Encourage the person to take time to meditate or pray, whether alone or together with you.
- Securing an appropriate cleric for the person.

Even if the person you are caring for does not share your own spiritual beliefs, he or she still has beliefs, and you must respect that. Your role is to offer comfort and support, but not to quarrel with the person for whom you are caring or to strong-arm him or her into your way of thinking. Part of providing an open, compassionate environment is to create a sense of togetherness that will allow the ill person to make his or her own honest investigation of matters that are of great spiritual concern to him or her.

As mentioned earlier, when a seriously ill person needs to discuss spiritual matters that go beyond your ability to help, don't hesitate to secure the services of a spiritual professional. But be careful not to be pushy in doing this. A decision to summon a spiritual professional should be made by the seriously ill person alone.

When you do not have adequate training in spiritual matters, a qualified cleric is needed to

- Guide the person's thinking in unfamiliar territory
- Ask proactive, searching questions
- Answer tough questions such as "Why me?" or "How can God let this happen to me?"
- Provide a symbolic presence of God, and offer the calming reassurance that God is control, and looks after his own
- Provide support by showing unconditional love
- Provide knowledge to help increase understanding of the unknown and afterlife, addressing anxieties and fears

- Help the person assess his or her expectations for himself or herself, his or her relationships with others, and his or her relationship with God

Certain times are crucial times when you may need to seek a spiritual leader to help someone who is seriously ill:

- When he or she desires to receive prayer or a blessing
- When pastoral counseling is required
- Immediately before serious surgery
- Immediately after an unsuccessful operation
- Soon after a negative diagnosis
- When a serious health problem recurs
- When the person needs to prepare himself or herself to face death
- When alienated family members whose estrangement concerns the ill person must be reconciled

Your faithful companionship, unlimited compassion, and unconditional acceptance are essential for you to provide the effective spiritual support that a seriously ill person requires. To the best of your ability, provide all the help you can offer, and be ready to call for the aid of a knowledgeable spiritual leader at any time that is appropriate.

59

Responding to Strong Feelings

Holding in creates horrid poisons
which wear us out before our time.
—ROBERTSON DAVIES

Those who are chronically ill, like most people, tend to be preoccupied with their own thoughts and feelings. It is highly recommended that you accept whatever feelings a sick person has, and that you encourage him or her to express them to you. An ill individual's willingness to share his or her strong feelings with you is an indication that you enjoy a close, warm, trusting relationship with him or her. And whenever you help an ailing person identify and understand his or her feelings, you help him or her become more comfortable and relaxed, because he or she knows that his or her feelings are accepted, and understood, by you.

It is essential that you acknowledge and respond to the feelings that are expressed to you. Empathize with the feelings of the ill person, but realize that if you identify too closely with these problems, you will be in danger of making the other person's problems your own problems. It is perfectly all right to share a person's feelings and problems, but it isn't a good idea to actually assume them.

Try to respond to the feelings that are being expressed, rather than concentrating only on the intellectual content of what the person is saying. It is important that you acknowledge and understand the feelings expressed, rather than merely listening to them; for example, you might say, "I can see you are upset and feeling frustrated because you don't seem to be getting any better." If you fail to respond adequately to the strong feelings expressed, you risk making the person feel frustrated, and you risk harming your relationship.

Strong feelings can create great discomfort and anxiety if held in and not aired. Because of this, it is desirable for you to help the person state such feelings immediately: "I get the sense that you're feeling extremely frustrated this morning. Why don't you tell me all about it? I'm here for you, and I'm ready to listen."

It's important to recognize that an ill person's strong feeling about something today may not be as strong tomorrow. (Strong feelings over something may be temporary rather than permanent; this is especially true if the person has had an opportunity to vent, fully letting off steam about something concerning him or her at the time.) But an interested, compassionate, and patient listener frequently alleviates feelings of discomfort and anxiety simply through his or her presence. It can't be stressed enough that empathetic listening, in and of itself, can be therapeutic.

After listening to a sick person utter his or her strong feelings about something bothering him or her, it is essential that you respond appropriately. One way is to simply restate the emotions expressed. If the person has been complaining about feeling helpless, you could say, "That sounds terrible—feeling helpless must be extremely frustrating. I share your concern." Or you could go a step further, after acknowledging that you have heard the person: "I can see you're hurting, and I'd like to help you if I can. What can I do to help you feel better?"

You can detect the intensity of emotions by paying close attention not only to the words being said but also to the volume and pitch of the person's voice and to facial expressions and overall body movement.

In addition to knowing what to say to a highly emotional person you're interacting with, it is equally important to know what not to say or do.

Things to Avoid Doing:
- Interrupting with your own comments—your thoughts and feelings are of little or no importance in such situations
- Showing any impatience or annoyance
- Looking amused, or kidding around to make light of the situation
- Looking bored or inattentive

- Trying to change the subject
- Responding emotionally yourself
- Acting shocked or disapproving

Things to Avoid Saying:
- "I want you to calm down and control yourself."
- "I'm not going to sit here and listen to you act like this."
- "I know exactly how you feel."
- "Relax—God will take care of you."
- * "You are talking pure nonsense—I want you to stop it right now."
- "I'm not going to listen to this; I'll be back later."
- "I don't consider you helpless, and I don't know where you get such a crazy idea."
- "I can see your medicine has got you riled up again."

Your goal when listening to a highly emotional person is to show compassion, and to act like a responsive sponge that is willing to absorb all the steam that is let off.

If emotional episodes become too frequent or too intense, consider obtaining the assistance of a health professional who is skilled in handling such situations. You can't expect to be all things to an ill person, and you need to know when it is best to call for competent help.

Appendix A

Symptoms of Caregiver Burnout

- Disrupted sleep patterns, including insomnia or habitually oversleeping; never feeling rested, even when the primary caregiver has managed to have a full night's sleep; sleep troubled by disturbing dreams or nightmares
- Altered eating patterns, including not being able to eat or overeating; significant weight gain or loss
- Increased sugar consumption or use of alcohol or drugs
- Increased smoking or strong desire to start again after having quit
- Frequent headaches or sudden onset of back pain.
- Increased reliance on over-the-counter pain remedies or prescribed drugs
- Irritability
- High levels of fear or anxiety
- Impatience
- The inability to handle one or more problems or crises
- Overreacting to commonplace accidents such as dropping a glass or misplacing something
- Overreacting to criticism

- Overreacting with anger toward a spouse, child, or older care recipient
- Alienation, even from those who offer relief and help
- Feeling emotional withdrawal
- Feeling trapped
- Thinking of disappearing or running away
- Not being able to laugh or feel joy
- Withdrawing from activities and the lives of others around the primary caregiver
- Feeling hopeless most of the time
- Loss of compassion
- Resenting the care recipient and/or the situation
- Neglecting or mistreating the care recipient
- Frequently feeling totally alone even though friends and family are present
- Wishing simply "to have the whole thing over with"
- Playing the "if only" games; saying over and over "If only this would happen" or "If only this hadn't happened"
- Loss of hope, purpose, and meaning
- Thinking of suicide as a means of escape

Adapted from "Preventing Caregiver Burnout," James R. Sherman, Ph.D., Pathway Books, 1994, pages 7, 11, and 12.

Appendix B

21 Stress Coping Methods for Caregivers

1. Have realistic expectations for yourself; be careful not to set them too high. Learn to accept what you cannot change, and focus only on the things you can change. You cannot give what you do not have.
2. Know your mental and physical limits. Be aware of your personal limitations regarding your availability to care for the ill person. You must know when to step back to recharge your energy batteries. (Be sure to explain your time and availability limitations to the person for whom you are caring.)
3. Maintain a positive attitude. View your caregiving role as an opportunity to develop a closer, deeper relationship with the person for whom you are caring, as well as a chance for you to grow as a person (try to associate frequently with people who have optimistic and positive outlooks on life).
4. Obtain advice on caregiving from experienced caregivers. Learn the various coping techniques in advance, rather than learning them the hard way through trial and error.
5. Explain the level of commitment required, and the accompanying time demands, to your family and friends to secure their support and understanding.

6. Share the caregiving duties and responsibilities as much as is possible and practical. You can't—and shouldn't—be the sole caregiver; try to have at least two other people help you.

7. Accept that as a caregiver, you need help; tell family and friends exactly what you will need. Write down the kinds of help you will require, and give copies to the appropriate people. Don't hesitate to ask for help whenever you need it; in addition, consider taking the other person to a daycare center several times a week.

8. Talk with an empathetic close friend or family member whenever things bother you. It is best to get it all out when you are feeling pressured, frustrated, or upset, rather than attempting to hold it all in. It is also a good idea to join a caregiver's support group.

9. Control the caregiving situation, rather than letting it control you; be proactive, rather than reactive, by securing agreement on ground rules of conduct when your caregiving begins.

10. Decide what is important, and set priorities. Focus on these priorities, and don't sweat the small stuff, wasting time and energy on minor matters.

11. Do your best to balance your previous life activities and routines with the newer demands of caregiving. You still have your own life to live.

12. Be empathetic with the other person and his or her problems, but refrain from making these problems your own. You can't—and shouldn't—own the ill person's problems; this is not only impossible, but unhealthy.

13. Keep your sense of humor; laugh big and often. A hearty laugh is therapeutic.

14. Develop the ability to temporarily block out problems by concentrating on something peaceful and enjoyable. Insist on some private time each day to take a mental vacation or to actually get away to do something you would like to do. It is essential to have something to look forward to at the end of each day or, at the least, each week. Learn to enjoy yourself without feeling guilty.

15. Engage in some mind-freeing activities daily, if at all possible. These activities vary by person, but commonly include listening to soothing sounds, such as music or ocean waves; viewing a sunset; gardening; taking a warm bath; getting a massage; playing a sport; doing something creative; or having a lighthearted talk with a friend.

16. Avail yourself of some reputable relaxation techniques, such as biofeedback, meditation, yoga, prayer, or deep-breathing exercises.

17. Keep mentally and physically fit:
    - Eat balanced, nutritious, stress-free meals at about the same time each day.
    - Get adequate sleep on a regular basis.
    - Take several brief rest periods daily.
    - See your doctor promptly when you need to.
    - Schedule periodic medical examinations.
    - Beware of too much self-medication (e.g., taking tranquilizers).

- Get lots of exercise regularly.

18. Identify the main things that cause you to feel stressed, and develop coping measures for them. Listen to your body; be alert to the physical and mental warning signs it gives you.

19. Learn to say no to excessive or unreasonable demands, whether made by the ill person or by others.

20. Encourage the ill person to do as many things for himself or herself as he or she can without overdoing it.

21. Know ahead of time what to say or do when your patience becomes exhausted by the ill person's excessive demands or verbal abuse. On such occasions, it is best to simply say, "I'm sorry—I need to leave now, but I'll be back later"; this approach is preferable to your remaining on the scene and showing anger or, worse yet, saying something in the heat of the moment that you'll regret later. Naturally, if the unacceptable behavior persists, you will need to confront the ill person to discuss what kinds of behavior are appropriate and inappropriate.

About the Author

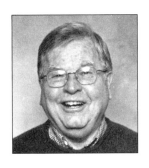

D r. Walter St. John is a retired college professor and administrator who lives with his wife in Old Town, Maine.

He taught interpersonal communications courses for more than twenty years and has presented communications workshops throughout the United States and Canada. He has hands-on experience with disabled veterans, multihandicapped youth, and Special Olympics participants, and he has written widely in the field of communications. His research for this book included consultations with numerous health care professionals.

Dr. St. John received his bachelor's degree from the University of Arizona, with a major in communications. Subsequently, he earned his doctorate from the University of Southern California, with a major in management and a minor in counseling.